THE VEGETARIAN Female

ANIKA AVERY-GRANT, RD

AVERY PUBLISHING
Garden City Park • New

D1360281

The dietary and nutritional information, procedures, and recommendations that are presented in this book are based on the research, training, and personal and professional experiences of the author, and are true and complete to the best of the author's knowledge. This book is intended as an informative guide. It is not intended to replace or countermand the advice given by a health-care professional. Because each person and each situation is unique, the publisher urges the reader to consult with a health-care professional before making any decisions or following any recommendations where there is a question regarding appropriateness.

The publisher does not advocate the use of any particular dietary regimen or supplement program, but believes that the information presented in the book should be available to the public. The author and publisher are not responsible for any adverse effects or consequences resulting from the use of any of the suggestions in this book. Please feel free to consult a physician or other qualified health professional.

Cover designer: Phaedra Mastrocola
Editor: Helene Ciaravino
Typesetter: Liz Johnson
Cover Photo Credit: PhotoDisc, Inc.
Printer: Paragon Press, Honesdale, PA

Avery Publishing Group, Inc.
120 Old Broadway
Garden City Park, NY 11040
1–800–548–5757
www.averypublishing.com

Library of Congress Cataloging-in-Publication Data

Avery-Grant, Anika L.
    The vegetarian female : a guide to a healthier diet for women
of all ages / by Anika L. Avery-Grant.
    p. cm.
    Includes bibliographical references and index.
    ISBN 0–89529–840–6
    1. Vegetarianism.   2. Women—Nutrition.   I. Title.
TX392.A94   1999
613.2'62'082—dc21   98–28316
                                                     CIP

Printed in the United States of America

10 9 8 7 6 5 4 3 2 1

Contents

PART THREE
THE VEGETARIAN ADVANTAGE OVER CHRONIC DISEASE

PART FOUR
THE TRANSITION TO A PLANT-BASED DIET

*This book is dedicated to the females in my life:
my mom, Ms. Avery; my grandmother, Mrs. Giddings;
my grandmother, Ms. Grier; my sister, Siena;
my Aunt Marilyn; my cousin, Siena;
and my two second cousins, Jasmine and Nilajah.*

Acknowledgments

To God be the glory. I would like to extend thanks to all of my family and friends who have supported and encouraged me throughout the writing of this book. My deepest gratitude is extended to my husband Mark, my mother Eleanor Avery, and my sister Siena. I would also like to thank my brothers Jelon and Ekene for their support. Last, but not least, I would like to thank Avery Publishing Group for even considering my work. A very special thanks goes to Rudy Shur and my editor Helene Ciaravino and to all the others for their hard work and wonderful ideas in making this book what it is today.

Codes and Abbreviations

g	gram(s)
hr	hour(s)
IU	international unit(s)
lb	pound(s)
mcg	microgram(s)
mg	milligram(s)
min	minute(s)
oz	ounce(s)
qt	quart(s)
tbsp	tablespoon(s)
tsp	teaspoon(s)
+	plus; and greater
>	greater than
<	less than

Preface

I have been a vegetarian since birth. My mother decided to follow a vegetarian diet when her first child was born. She followed through with her desire and raised all four of her children as vegetarians. We were lacto-ovo-vegetarians throughout my childhood years, and then made the change to veganism when I began my mid-teens.

My interest in nutrition, health, and cooking started at a very early age and continued to grow as I read more and more about how health is directly affected by the foods we eat. I began to realize that a vegetarian diet is an important asset to disease prevention and health maintenance. It followed that I chose to enter the field of nutrition, for it would provide me with the knowledge I needed to help others make healthy life choices.

I began my studies in nutrition with many misconceptions concerning what people think about healthy diets and vegetarianism. It didn't take long for me to learn that not all people feel that "health" and "vegetarianism" belong in the same sentence. In fact, many think that the two terms are directly opposed to one another. I was rather perplexed and disappointed when I realized that the majority of the questions I expected to be answered about vegetarianism during my college years would have to be researched and discovered on my own.

Nonetheless, my experiences and research helped me to understand several things. First, even though a lifetime vegetarian, I have had a lot to learn about vegetarianism. Second, society, as a whole, believes in many false myths and assumptions about vegetarian diets. Third, the benefits of vegetarianism extend far past personal health. Fourth, few health professionals can dispense accurate information regarding vegetarianism and following a vegetarian diet. Finally, I learned that there is a definite need for a comprehensive guidebook that promotes a vegan diet and gives clear-cut, practical advice on healthfully following a vegan lifestyle. It is as a result of these conclusions that I felt compelled to write *The Vegetarian Female*.

Introduction

Maybe you are a vegetarian or are considering becoming one. Maybe you just want to eat more vegetarian meals, or investigate the whole concept of veganism. Perhaps you are worried about your family's wellness and are looking for a healthy lifestyle change. Perhaps you are concerned about the environment and the way our factory farm animals are treated, and you want to do something about it. If you find yourself in any one of these categories, then *The Vegetarian Female* is definitely for you.

The Vegetarian Female promotes women's health through education on vegetarianism, and veganism in particular. The message is easy: you can enhance wellness and contribute to a kinder world by following a vegan diet. But learning to manage a healthy diet without the old American staples of meat and dairy can be very challenging. So, I offer you specific guidelines and sincere encouragement.

Part One of *The Vegetarian Female* discusses the definitions and history of vegetarianism, identifies influential vegetarian women, and studies the benefits of eating *no* animal products. Part Two explains how to attain a balanced diet without animal products, and how to plan that diet according to the different stages of a female's life. Part Three discusses prevention of the major chronic diseases and disorders that afflict many women, including information on how vegetarianism can help. Lastly, Part Four helps to guide and support you through the transition to a plant-based diet, if you are just deciding to make the change. It also contains useful facts on purchasing, storing, and preparing vegan foods.

The Vegetarian Female is not just a book about diet and eating. It deals with the whole woman. This text encourages you to integrate physical activity, mental stability, emotional balance, and spiritual health with a vegetarian diet, with the aim of achieving a disease-free and joyous life. In addition, I not only address environmental damage, world hunger, and animal cruelty, but explain how we can help to alleviate these horrors. The way you eat can make a positive difference in your own personal life and the lives of those around you.

This book is a guide for females, written by a female who believes in the power of choice. The choices we make can improve, enrich, and nurture life, or they can destroy life. You will find that upon reading this book, you will be more conscientious about food consumption, current health issues, our environment, and its creatures. *The Vegetarian Female* will help you take a large step toward a better you and a better world.

Part One

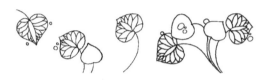

Introduction to Vegetarianism

In the hands of women rests a great responsibility,
for the choices they make will either give life
or take it away.

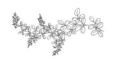 # Chapter 1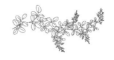

Vegetarian Females—
A Healthful Sisterhood

"Free at last, free at last, thank God Almighty, I'm free at last." These were some of the final public words of Martin Luther King, Jr., Nobel-prize winner and nonviolent civil rights leader. And these words are poignantly carved into the monument at the site where King lies in Atlanta, Georgia. They inspire us to reach for something better. Today, Caretta Scott King, wife of Martin Luther King, Jr., continues to march toward a more peaceful, just world. She does so not only by promoting the civil rights philosophies of her husband, but also by following a meatless diet that includes no animal products. Mrs. King and two of her children are vegans who believe that vegetarianism is a logical extension of nonviolence and personal development.

According to a 1992 survey performed by *Vegetarian Times* magazine, over 12.4 million Americans consider themselves vegetarian. The magazine also reported that of its over 326,000 (and growing) subscribers, 89 percent are females. Furthermore, in 1994, the Vegetarian Resource Group took a nationwide poll of 1,978 men and women over 18 years of age. From this representative sample, it was concluded that up to half of a million individuals in this country may actually be vegan—that is, they consume absolutely no animal products at all. These numbers undoubtedly continue to grow as vegetarianism becomes more accepted as a healthier way to eat.

There is an increasing body of evidence that suggests that vegetarian women are healthier than nonvegetarian women. Modern research finds that, when they are compared with their meat-eating counterparts, vegetarian females have lower incidences of heart disease, breast cancer, colon cancer, lung cancer, osteoporosis, diabetes, and obesity! A 1994 study on vegetarian and nonvegetarian women, performed by Knutsen and colleagues and published in the *American Journal of Clinical Nutrition,* found that the vegetarian diet reduces the incidence of chronic disease, the amount of medication taken, the health services used, and medical-care costs.

The greater the amount of research that is conducted concerning vegetarianism, the more convincing it is that a vegetarian diet is not only a health-enhancing, disease-inhibiting diet, but a compassionate, economical, earth-preserving diet that is not difficult to properly balance. It's no wonder that many people admit to either wanting to become vegetarian or wanting to eat more vegetarian meals! Yet before we begin the discussion on present-day women's health issues and all of the benefits of vegetarianism, it is helpful to take a few steps back and look at the meaning and the history of vegetarianism.

THE DEFINITION OF A VEGETARIAN

Some dictionaries define a vegetarian as one who abstains from all animal flesh and lives on vegetables, eggs, milk, and dairy products. This is a poor definition indeed, for it actually refers to only one type of vegetarian—the lacto-ovovegetarian. It is more accurate to define a vegetarian simply as one who abstains from all animal flesh.

There are three general types of vegetarians. *Lacto-ovovegetarians* consume eggs, milk, other dairy products, vegetables, fruits, nuts/seeds, grains, and legumes. *Lactovegetarians* follow a diet that includes the same foods as the lacto-ovovegetarians, but without the eggs. Finally, *vegans* eat a strictly plant-based diet, avoiding all flesh foods and animal products, including both eggs and dairy products. (Some vegans consider honey to be an animal product, as well.) There are vegetarians who extend their convictions to other areas of life and will not purchase items such as lard-containing bathing soap, leather shoes and clothing, coats made with animal hair, etc.

The origin of the term *vegetarian* is quite fascinating. The word is derived from the Latin word *vegetus,* meaning "whole, sound, fresh, and lively." Consequently, the ancient Latin word *homo-vegetus* refers to a mentally and physically vigorous person. How did the context and meaning evolve to its present use? Well, perhaps we should consider the phrase, "You are what you eat." Most people cannot deny that whole grains, fruits, vegetables, legumes, nuts, and seeds have been known to promote both physical and mental health. Simply stated, vegetarian foods are whole, sound, fresh, and life-enhancing. In my opinion, flesh foods cannot be defined in the same manner.

SOME HISTORY ON VEGETARIANISM

The lifestyle of vegetarianism can be traced back over millennia. In some cases, vegetarianism has been an act of compassion. In other cases, it has been a holy obligation. Whatever the reason, vegetarianism tends to affect the body, mind, and spirit.

Ancient Roots

Vegetarianism, as a chosen way of life, is said to have been instituted by Pythagoras of Samos, a Greek philosopher of the sixth century B.C. Because of his compassion for animals, Pythagoras resolved to nourish himself on a meatless diet. He is quoted as saying, "As long as man continues to be the ruthless destroyer of lower living beings, he will never know health or peace. For as long as men massacre animals, they will kill each other. Indeed, he who sows the seed of murder and pain cannot reap joy and love." Many other philosophers, including Epicurus and Plutarch, followed Pythagoras' example and lived vegetarian lifestyles. These latter philosophers apparently subscribed to vegetarianism because of their belief in the transmigration of souls, or reincarnation.

The belief in the transmigration of souls is also embedded in the philosophies of Hinduism. The Hindu way of life actually dates back more than 3,000 years and is considered one of the world's oldest religions. A vegetarian diet is followed in some of the Hindu castes (classes of Hindu society) because of the people's unwillingness to destroy living things. In the Hindu culture, many animals and plants are considered sacred. The cow is held especially sacred, so even those castes that do not adhere to vegetarianism still refrain from eating beef.

While both the above-mentioned Greek philosophers and many early followers of Hinduism certainly promoted the vegetarian diet, it was truly established even long before. The implementation of vegetarianism can be found in Genesis, the first book of the Old Testament, which dates back to 4004 B.C. Genesis 1:29 states, "And God said, Behold I have given you every herb bearing seed which is upon the face of all the earth, and every tree, in which is the fruit of a tree yielding seed; to you it shall be for meat." Also, Genesis 3:18 proclaims, ". . . and thou shalt eat the herb of the field." These verses reveal that grains, fruits, nuts, seeds, and vegetables have been given to us as the ideal diet from the beginning of time. And a diet of plant foods is not only good for humans, but is also beneficial to our planet and the animals that inhabit it.

Today's Vegetarian Movement

Despite its ancient roots, the vegetarian movement did not develop in the United States until the nineteenth century. It actually grew out of the dietary teachings of several individuals, including: Reverend Sylvester Graham, the inventor of the graham cracker; Antonio Cocchi, the Keeper of the Duke of Tuscany's museum and a Fellow of the Royal Society of London; William A. Alcott, a physician and author of *Vegetable Diet: As Sanctioned by Medical Men and by Experience in All Ages;* Dr. John Kellogg, well-known for his breakfast cereals; Ellen G. White, the founder of the Seventh-day Adventist Church; and others.

The vegetarian movement has gained enormous strides over the years, as evidenced by the increasing number of individuals becoming vegetarians. This progress is primarily due to a number of books that were published in the latter half of the twentieth century and that have strongly promoted the vegetarian diet. Among these books are Frances Moore Lappé's *Diet for a Small Planet;* John Robbins' *May All Be Fed: Diet for a New World;* and numerous vegetarian recipe books.

In addition, the establishment of several vegetarian interest groups and organizations around the world has played a large part in strengthening the vegetarian movement and stretching its tendrils far and wide. These organizations are committed to educating the public about the benefits of a vegetarian lifestyle. They also provide support groups for those who are just making the dietary decision, as well as for those who have followed vegetarianism for years. From the Vegan Society based in Australia to the European Vegetarian Union, from the People for the Ethical Treatment of Animals (PETA) in the United States to the Brighton Vegetarian and Vegan Society in the United Kingdom, many individuals are doing their part to make sure that the vegetarian movement continues to grow.

Furthermore, modern research strongly supports that vegetarianism promotes health and wellness by preventing chronic disease. As a result, organizations such as the vegetarian chapters of the American Dietetic Association and the National Institute for Cancer Research promote a plant-based diet. In Part Three of this book, you will read about specific chronic diseases and how vegetarianism helps to prevent their onset and treat their effects.

The increasingly researched and popular soybean should not go unnoticed when it comes to promoting the vegetarian lifestyle. The soybean has probably done more than any other plant food to encourage vegetarianism, or at least a primarily plant-based diet. Soybean products have been getting a lot of press. According to the 1997 National Report on consumer attitudes about nutrition from the United Soybean Board, 59 percent of Americans believe soy is healthy and 70 percent say that they have tried some type of soy product. One in three consumers who eat soy products at least once per week reported that a magazine or news article influenced them to incorporate soy into their meals.

The vegetarian movement should only expect to expand as more and more dietary research from the medical, environmental, and animal rights communities is conducted. These groups are constantly finding new indications that the health of our bodies, the preservation of our natural resources, the solution to world hunger, and the treatment of our animals can all be addressed through a vegetarian diet.

VEGETARIANISM'S FAMOUS FEMALES

It is important to realize that women have played an important role in the promotion of vegetarianism. Many women spread health and compassion within their own homes through vegetarian ideals and cooking. And the following paragraphs highlight two influential females whose names and work you very well may recognize.

Ellen G. White

Few historians consider Ellen G. White (1827–1915) to be one of the founding mothers of the vegetarian movement in the United States. However, I find that her teachings and writings clearly identify her as a strong advocate for vegetarianism. As the founder of Seventh-day Adventism, whose followers serve as the most researched group of vegetarians today, Mrs. White has had great impact on the advancement of vegetarianism in this country.

Mrs. White was born Ellen G. Harmon on November 26, 1827 at Gorham, Maine. At the tender age of 17, she had a religious experience and began to write and to preach. One of the foundational truths that she found revealed to her was the importance of following a vegetarian diet. In one of her books entitled *Ministry of Healing,* Ellen White states:

> *Those who eat flesh are but eating grains and vegetables at second hand; for the animal receives from these things the nutrition that produces growth. The life that was in the grains and vegetables passes into the eater. We receive it by eating the flesh of the animal.*

How much better to get it direct, by eating the food that God pro-
vided for our use!

In the same book, White writes:

> *. . . Flesh was never the best food; but its use is now double*
> *objectionable, since disease in animals is so rapidly increasing.*
> *Those who use flesh foods little know what they are eating. Often if*
> *they could see the animals when living, and know the quality of the*
> *meat they eat, they would turn from it with loathing.*

The lifestyle promoted by Ellen White not only includes vegetarianism, but also many other health-enhancing practices. It calls for abstinence from tobacco, drugs, alcohol, and caffeine. Regular exercise and adequate sleep are strongly encouraged. Seventh-day Adventists also reserve the Sabbath —from sunset Friday to sunset Saturday—as a holy day of rest, relaxation, and rejuvenation of the body, mind, and spirit. Indeed, the writings of Ellen White have not only advanced the cause of vegetarianism, but that of over-all healthy living.

Frances Moore Lappé

Nearly 100 years after Ellen G. White wrote the above statements, another female started writing about the benefits of vegetarianism and the adverse effects of a meat-based diet. Frances Moore Lappé was born in 1944. She attended a small Quaker college and graduated in 1966. Then Lappé attend-ed graduate school at the University of California at Berkeley, where she devoted herself to the study of community organizing. Her dissatisfaction with humankind's suffering led her to make a very important decision in the spring of 1969. In her book, *Diet for a Small Planet,* Lappé reveals how she decided not to try to "change the world" until she understood the moti-vations behind her own choices and until she figured out what she could do to end avoidable suffering.

That decision, Lappé says, was the most important one of her life, causing her to drop out of graduate school at the age of 25, and eventual-ly leading Lappé into a quest to find the source of and solution to world hunger. Her research resulted in an astounding and admirable conclusion: ". . . if I could write up the facts about how land and grain are wasted through a fixation of meat production, and could demonstrate that there are delicious alternatives, I could get people to question the economic ground rules that create such irrational patterns of resource use." And she did.

Frances Moore Lappé's first edition of *Diet for a Small Planet* (1971), which sold more than 3 million copies, rocked America. In her work, Lappé explains the antagonism that vegetarians have endured: ". . . anyone who questioned the American diet's reliance on beef—since cattle are the most wasteful converters of grain to meat—was perceived as challenging the American way of life (especially, when that someone came from Fort Worth, Texas—'Cowtown, USA')." She also states, ". . . the notion that human beings could do well without meat was heretical. Today, the medical establishment acknowledges the numerous benefits of eating low on the food chain." Lappé's facts on how meat production harms our economy, our planet, and our health have enlightened countless Americans.

Did You Know About These Vegetarians?

Many women have played enormous roles in the promotion of the vegetarian lifestyle. For example, Virginia Messina, MPH, RD, is a registered dietitian who has accomplished much work in the area of vegetarian nutrition. She was coauthor of the 1997 American Dietetic Association's position paper on vegetarian diets. In addition, Messina has served as an editor for a number of vegetarian publications, including *Issues in Vegetarian Dietetics*, and is currently senior editor of the *Vegetarian Nutrition and Health Letter*. She is cofounder of *Vegetarian Nutrition: An International Journal*, which is a peer-reviewed journal. Finally, Mrs. Messina has coauthored several books: *The Vegetarian Way; The Dietitian's Guide to Vegetarian Diets: Issues and Applications; The Simple Soybean and Your Health; The Vegetarian No-Cholesterol Barbecue Book;* and *The Vegetarian No-Cholesterol Family Style Cookbook.*

Dietitian Reed Mangels, PhD, RD, and Debra Wasserman authored two books on the vegan diet. These works are entitled *Simply Vegan* and *Vegan Handbook*. Both books provide the vegan with excellent nutrition and health information, as well as plenty of recipes. Wasserman has also authored *Conveniently Vegan*.

Suzanne Havala, RD, LDN, FADA, is also a dietitian and a primary author of the American Dietetic Association's position paper on vegetarian diets. She is the Nutrition Adviser for the Vegetarian Resource Group and is on the editorial advisory board of the *Vegetarian Times* magazine. Havala has authored a book entitled *Simple, Lowfat, and Vegetarian.*

Actually, any woman who follows a vegetarian diet is doing her part in advocating this way of life. Vegetarianism has grasped women of all nationalities and backgrounds, and has brought them to a common ground built on respect for their bodies and their health, the health of their families, compassion for animals, and care for this earth.

Ms. Victoria Lidiard was one of the last woman suffragettes to be jailed while fighting for a woman's right to vote. She was also a vegetarian for ninety years. She died in 1992, at the age of 103. Though Lidiard did not go down in history as an advocate for vegetarianism, her long life on a vegetarian diet is evidence that she helped to advance this cause, too.

It is no surprise that vegetarianism has reached celebrity heights. Many women who are constantly in the public eye have found that a vegetarian diet can help them control their weight and can keep them feeling and looking healthy and vibrant. Let me throw out a few names. Phylicia Rashad and Lisa Bonet from *The Cosby Show* are vegetarians, while their fellow cast member Sabrina LeBeauf is a vegan. Meredith Baxter from *Family Ties* is a vegetarian, and *Roseanne's* Sarah Gilbert is a vegan. Lindsay Wagner, the star of the *Bionic Woman* series, has authored a vegan cookbook, *The High Road to Health.* Wagner was the first female celebrity who I heard was a vegan. I was thrilled and impressed with her book and her promotion of such a life-giving diet. And even Lisa from *The Simpsons,* a popular comedy-cartoon series, has decided to take a lonely but firm stand for vegetarianism!

Singer and actress Vanessa Williams, among whose films include *Eraser* and *Dance With Me,* is vegetarian. So are singer and actress Kim Bassinger, who starred in *Batman* and *L.A. Confidential,* as well as other films, and actress Alicia Silverstone from such movies as *Clueless* and *Batman and Robin.* Models Christie Brinkley and Yasmin LeBon have found a vegetarian diet to be ideal for them. And vegetarianism has entered the music world: Olivia Newton John is a vegetarian, and K.D. Lang and Heather Small are vegan vegetarians.

Many meat-eaters believe that of all people, those involved in sports cannot support themselves on a vegetarian, much less a vegan, diet. Well, just look at vegan Ruth Heidrich, who is a three-time Ironman finisher and a marathoner. Heidrich is the President of the Vegetarian Society of Honolulu, Hawaii. And consider vegan Romy Korz, a soloist ballerina with the nascent Los Angeles Ballet. Debbie Lawrence is the world-record holder for the women's 5K racewalk event and a vegetarian. Finally, Nicky Cole, a vegetarian, was the first woman to walk to the North Pole. These amazing women are proof that a plant-based diet is more than adequate when it comes to enhancing life.

From royalty such as Queen Sofia of Spain, to politicians such as Anne Campbell, to President Bill Clinton's daughter Chelsea, to folk like me and maybe even you, women around the world are subscribing to vegetarianism. The seed that we plant will spring up into a beautiful tree that will yield many fruits, and in these fruits will be more seeds. So the cycle continues to bear life, health, and happiness.

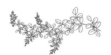 # Chapter 2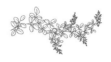

Why *Not* Vegetarianism?

I have been a vegetarian all of my life, so I am quite used to the common question: "Why vegetarianism?" As an adolescent growing up, I would simply say, "Because of my religion." As a college student, I would answer, "Because of my health and my religion." When I graduated from college, I would respond, "Because of my health, animal welfare, and my religion." It was not until I started working on this book that I found the perfect answer, "Why not vegetarianism?" After all, it makes perfect sense.

The most common question posed to those who follow a meatless diet is, "Why did you become a vegetarian?" Each vegetarian has his or her individual response, but the reasons generally fall into one or more of the following categories: compassion for animals; health and physical fitness; ethical, philosophical, religious, and/or spiritual convictions; solution to world hunger; ecological and environmental issues; and concern for economics and medical costs. Ultimately, most of the answers boil down to the desire to enhance life by choosing a diet that promotes life.

When meat-eaters defend their meat-eating, they usually respond by saying that meat tastes good, that it contains many nutrients, that our ancestors ate meat, or simply that we are meant to eat meat. Notice that much of the drive behind these answers is different than the motivations behind the dietary decisions of vegetarians.

I'd like you to ask yourself a question: What price am I willing to pay for what I choose to eat? Very few of us ever take the time to learn about how our particular lifestyles impact the world around us. So few of us realize that the diets we choose can either help to end world hunger or contribute to broadening its boundaries. Our dietary choices can encourage cruelty to animals or work to alleviate suffering. They can help save our natural resources or they can promote the rapid destruction of nature. Our food habits even either save or spend government dollars in medical care. Indeed, as intelligent human beings, we should take the time to count the costs and benefits of what we eat.

THE CREATURES OF THE EARTH

It is no secret that food animals are subjected to terrible conditions, but most of us do not want to be bothered with knowing the ugly details because knowledge brings responsibility. Yet lack of knowledge never changed the truth. And the truth is that most animals raised for human consumption in industrialized nations suffer a frighteningly cruel and unnatural existence. Consider this passage from Joan Dye Gussow's article titled "Ecology and vegetarian considerations: does environmental responsibility demand the elimination of livestock?". Gussow's source for these facts is Mason J. Singer's *Animal Factories,* which describes the physical abuse of hogs raised for food.

> *The hogs' hooves are often damaged and their bones deformed. The hog factories could be redesigned, but the preferred solution is to redesign the factory hog: cut off the tail, regulate the females' estrus with drugs, suppress disease with antibiotics, and relocate the boar's penis surgically so that the boar becomes a "sidewinder" that cannot breed but can mount and thus "identify" the sows ready for artificial insemination.*

Almost any human confronted with this knowledge is shocked and appalled. And what about those countless cattle? In *The New Vegetarian,* author Gary Null explains how the steer is taken away from its mother almost immediately after birth. He is placed on a drug-filled "calf starter ration" that actually causes the creature to have less energy. Once he matures, the steer is often fed grass and processed feed that has been supplemented with growth-inducing drugs and antibiotics.

Jeremy Rifkin, in his book *Beyond Beef: The Rise and Fall of the Cattle Culture,* expounds on the horrors of how young male calves are treated. He reveals that they are castrated with the intention to keep them "docile" while alive to provide a better quality of beef. In addition, these animals are dehorned "with a chemical paste that burns out the roots of their horns" to avoid injury to each other. The cows are fed to reach 1,100 pounds. Now fully grown steers, large numbers of these animals are crammed into truck trailers. The trip to the slaughterhouse is a disgustingly difficult one for the steers; some can't move at all, while many others fall and are trampled. As a result, there are a lot of severe injuries, such as painful breaks in the pelvises and legs.

We anger at the slaughter of elephants for their ivory. We are saddened by the realization that many species of whales are on the brink of extinction because of humankind's greed. We get aggravated when illegal poachers kill protected animals in our wildlife sanctuaries. We are disgusted with the common abuse of cats and dogs by seemingly heartless and apathetic individuals. Yet when it comes to feeling for the animals who are bred and/or confined purely for the purpose of putting food on our plates, we do our best to turn a deaf ear. In fact, we continue to live as if the slaughterhouses that alter animals instead of altering the methods of treating animals never exist.

Consider these additional facts concerning the consequences of a food industry that relies on animal and marine life:

- Animals raised for food must be docked, debeaked, dehorned, and drugged because of their extremely confined conditions.

- Bovine spongiform encephalopathy (BSE), more commonly known as mad cow disease, is an incurable dementia that has killed 160,000 British cows since 1985. This disease is linked to the feeding of cow remains to livestock—an appalling and disgusting practice, as cows are natural herbivores.

- Thousands of sharks, turtles, and billfish are killed in the process of catching tuna.

- Twenty pounds or more of other sea creatures are caught for every pound of shrimp sold.

- The World Conservation Union lists 1,081 fish world-wide as being either threatened or endangered.

The figures are alarming. Yet most humans excuse their apathy toward creatures used for food by saying, "One person making a change is not going to do anything. Those slaughterhouses and commercial fishing vessels aren't just in existence because of me. They provide food for millions of people." Yes, they do provide food for millions, but a plant-based diet could provide food for millions more. The politics of meat production are driven by the same force that drives capitalism—supply and demand. If there was no demand for meat, there would be no need to supply it. So the ball bounces right back into each person's court. Things are going to have to change, individual by individual. Never underestimate the power of one. Throughout human history, our world has been affected countless times by one.

A simple question may help you to achieve a clearer perspective: Why should I eat animals when it is more humane to eat a plant-based diet? People who choose a vegetarian diet out of concern for animal welfare show respect and compassion for life, and they put into practice one of the greatest moral principles, "Do unto others as you would have them do unto you." If all people could see the despicable conditions and treatment that food animals endure to supply the carnivorous American diet, I am willing to bet that most of them would turn away from meat-eating in disgust and grief.

BASIC HEALTH

Health is actually the most common reason why people go vegetarian. And well it should be, since heart disease and cancer, America's number one and number two killers respectively, have strong correlations to dietary lifestyle habits. It is estimated that over 900,000 Americans die every year from cardiovascular disease (CVD), and 500,000 die from cancer. Think about it. Every day, people—mothers, fathers, sisters, brothers, relatives, friends— are dying from these diseases that often are directly linked to what they choose to eat.

The familiar saying, "what goes around comes around," is true and applicable in this instance. We senselessly and cruelly kill animals for food and, in turn, the consumption of their flesh can contribute to our own suffering from illness. In "An Opinion on the Global Impact of Meat Consumption," an article published in the *American Journal of Clinical Nutrition,* author Stephen Lewis eloquently states, "While millions of human beings go hungry for lack of adequate grain, millions more of the industrial world die from disease caused by an excess of grain-fed animal flesh, especially beef, in their diets."

Meat-eaters are at higher risk of and have higher incidences of: heart-disease; various cancers, including colon, lung, stomach, and breast cancers; high blood pressure; obesity; osteoporosis; diabetes; gallbladder disease; kidney stones; diverticular disease; and food-borne illnesses. Cancers, in particular, are linked not just to the consumption of high-fat, high-cholesterol, fiberless foods, but to the contaminants contained within them. These contaminants include drugs, hormones, and pesticides that can be found in flesh foods. In *Diet for a Small Planet,* Frances Moore Lappé reveals that meat, poultry, and fish contain more than double the amount of chlorinated pesticides than dairy products, and thirteen times more than grains, cereals, leafy and root vegetables, and fruit. All of these factors play a hand in producing what could be considered toxic food.

ETHICS AND AESTHETICS

Ethics are moral principles by which a person is guided, and ethical vegetarians are seriously opposed to the destruction of animals for food. They believe that humans should respect all life, human and other, and therefore reason that an individual can receive a proper diet without consuming other creatures. This motivation can be related to compassion for animals and to religious/spiritual convictions.

Aesthetics refers to an appreciation of beauty and art, and people who are vegetarian for aesthetic purposes believe that eating the dead corpse of an animal creates and maintains no beauty. They believe that people try to conceal the true origin of certain cuts of meat by assigning fancy names to them. For example, Rocky Mountain oysters are actually pig testicles. Decorative names like sirloin, brisket, and escargot simply make flesh sound elegant. Aesthetes find that fruits, nuts, and vegetables need no concealment and can be eaten in their fresh and natural state. They also claim that if people had to kill, cut, and clean their own meat, many would abstain from flesh foods because the smell and the sight of a corpse is so repulsive.

RELIGION AND SPIRITUALITY

Some vegetarians make their dietary decisions according to religious beliefs. For example, such vegetarians who are Jewish or Christian can find instruction in the Bible's Book of Genesis. According to that text, our ancestors' first and original diet was a vegan diet. The diet was given to the first humans in Eden, and even after they were driven from Eden, they were still instructed to consume only plant foods. According to sacred writ, we are to return to what we were first meant to be. The Bible terms it "the restitution of all things" in Acts 3:21.

Many religions follow doctrines that teach against the consumption of animal flesh. For example, the Seventh-day Adventists promote a meatless diet. Hinduism is actually the largest religion that mandates vegetarianism. Hindus believe in the reincarnation of souls in many life forms and, thus, animals are considered sacred. Jainist monks are one of the few religious groups who follow a strict vegan diet. There are also followers of Mormonism, Christianity, and Judaism who believe that animals do not exist for human consumption. Many members of these religions find that the horrible treatment of animals involved in the meat industry is not consistent with their religious values and convictions of being kind and compassionate.

Health of body and mind is another reason why certain religions require vegetarianism. A physically healthy body and mind is open to the influences of the Spirit of God. By following the healthiest of diets—a non-flesh diet—a person can attain optimal health and, therefore, enhanced spirituality.

ACTION AGAINST WORLD HUNGER

It was Frances Moore Lappé who first addressed the startling statistics concerning how much it actually costs, in human lives, to eat a meat-based diet. While starvation is rampant throughout many countries, including Ethiopia, Somalia, the Sudan, India, and others, Americans are actually throwing away enormous amounts of money and resources just to support meat-eating.

Lappé's *Diet for a Small Planet* reveals that it takes approximately 16 pounds of grain to produce just 1 pound of feedlot beef, while it takes only 1 pound of grain to produce 1 pound of wholesome bread. In *Diet for a New America,* author John Robbins states that 1 billion, 300 million human beings could be fed by the grain and soybeans fed to livestock in the United States. Furthermore, Robbins reports that if Americans were to reduce their meat consumption by only 10 percent, 100 million people could be fed with the land, water, and energy freed from the decrease in breeding livestock.

Robbins' point is confirmed by the fact that only 20 percent of the corn grown in the United States is eaten by human beings, while 80 percent of the corn, 90 percent of the soy, and 95 percent of the oats grown in the United States is eaten by livestock. These statistics become much more significant when we realize that somewhere throughout the world, a child dies of starvation approximately every two seconds. What a waste of our natural resources and what a selfish way to live! Indeed, I must agree with this quote from Amato and Patridge's *The New Vegetarians: Promoting Health and Protecting Life:* "Feeding food that people can eat, such as grains and beans, to animals for slaughter is crazy when there are so many people starving."

While cutting the meat and eating vegetarian won't solve all of the complex world hunger problems, vegetarianism is definitely a major factor to be considered in alleviating hunger. In *Our Hungry Earth: The World Food Crisis,* author Lawrence Pringle writes, "If we have the good sense and the will to change to a less wasteful lifestyle, we will provide a new model for the millions of people who want to emulate us. And that, perhaps even more than surplus grain, will be a powerful force in our efforts to solve the world food crises." Every person makes a difference, and your example is as powerful a tool as any.

ECOLOGY AND THE ENVIRONMENT

Most people do not become vegetarians because of the beneficial effects vegetarianism has on our planet. Usually, it is only after someone becomes a vegetarian that they learn of the devastating, large-scale effects that meat production causes, and how unwisely our earth's resources are being used to promote a diet that feeds the few instead of the many. Consider these statistics, reported in John Robbins' book, *May All Be Fed: Diet for a New World:*

- On one acre of land, 20,000 pounds of potatoes can be grown, while only 165 pounds of beef can be produced.

- Half of the entire earth's land mass is used as grazing land for livestock. In the United States alone, 64 percent of the cropland produces livestock feed.

- More than 60 percent of the world's rangelands have been damaged by overgrazing during the past half-century. And in the western United States, 85 percent of the rangeland is being degraded by overgrazing. In fact, the most common cause of desertification—the process of land becoming arid and turning into desert, often due to land mismanagement or climate changes—is overgrazing.

- In the production of 1 pound of feedlot steak, 35 pounds of topsoil are lost.

- Five million acres of Central and South American rain forest are felled every year to create cattle pasture. In fact, cattle ranching has destroyed more Central American rain forest than any other activity. In Panama and Costa Rica, 70 percent of cleared forests are now pastures.

- It takes 25 gallons of water to produce 1 pound of wheat, while it takes 2,500 gallons of water to produce 1 pound of protein from beefsteak.

- Factory farms are the biggest contributors to polluted rivers and streams in the United States.

- In 1993, 1,785 bodies of water were polluted by feedlots in thirty-nine U.S. states.

Obviously, the meat industry has a terrible effect on the natural beauty and balance of our planet. If you are thinking about vegetarianism, keep

Table 2.1. National Medical-Care Cost

Disease	Total Cost, in billions of dollars	Cost Due to Meat Consumption, in billions of dollars
Hypertension	12.5	2.8–8.5
Heart Disease	40.4	9.5
Cancer	35.3	0.0–16.5
Diabetes	45.2	14.0–17.1
Gallbladder Disease	3.2	0.2–2.4
Obesity	4.4	1.9
Food-borne Illness	6.0	0.2–5.5
Total	**108.0**	**28.6–61.4**

these factors in mind. It is rewarding to know that when you give up animal foods, you stop contributing to a widespread abuse of the earth.

MONEY MATTERS

Only a few studies have compared the medical-care costs of meat-eaters with those of vegetarians, but the studies reveal that vegetarians have the advantage. Table 2.1 shows that consumption of a vegetarian diet alone can save as much as over $40 billion in national medical-care costs per year. The table compares the total medical-care cost with the amount of medical-care costs attributed largely to meat consumption. When you subtract the latter from the former, you realize how significant national savings would be if we all cut back on meat.

So if you are asked, "Why vegetarianism?", answer with a better question: "Why *not* vegetarianism?" By following a vegetarian lifestyle, the benefits gained by our bodies, our animals, our environment, and even our pocketbooks are clear. There are some questions in life that we never will be able to answer, and acceptance is all that we can achieve. But other things make perfect sense—like a vegetarian diet—and it's so nice to find and hold onto them.

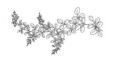 # Chapter 3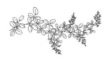

One Step Further— No Dairy, No Eggs

Colleen Brennan, a vegan dietitian, had written up two special tofu recipes for a cookbook that the staff at her facility was writing for the patients. She was surprised at the positive response she received from some of her coworkers. Some of them had actually tried the recipes. Colleen was even more elated when two coworkers came to her with questions, as they were thinking about becoming vegetarians and wanted more information. Colleen set up an appointment to meet one of these interested coworkers and his wife.

The couple was initially aiming to become lacto-ovovegetarians, but before the session with Colleen was over, they realized that a vegan diet was the way to go, for it insures a lower incidence of such health problems as foodborne illnesses and high cholesterol. The more they learned about the benefits of veganism and how simple it was to cook delicious vegan alternatives, the more excited they became. Today, the couple has committed themselves and their family to making the transition to a completely plant-based diet.

The choice to abstain from milk and eggs is difficult for most people to grasp, especially since we have been told over and over again that "milk does a body good" and that eggs are the perfect protein. The media constantly bombards us with the importance of these two items in our daily diet. Even most health professionals believe that a diet that excludes milk and eggs is an incomplete diet. But is the consumption of these foods absolutely necessary for health, and do they have the potential to increase your risk for illness? After reading this chapter, you be the judge.

MILK—THE PERFECT FOOD?

To be completely honest with you, milk is a perfect food. The problem comes when we add just two more words to the previous phrase: . . . *for humans.* Milk is a perfect food for baby calves. Unfortunately, many calves get very little, if any, of it. Too often, their mothers are milk machines and, later, hamburger meat for the human population in industrialized countries. Cow's milk definitely is not for baby humans, or any humans for that matter. The consumption of cow's milk causes newborn infants to suffer from intestinal bleeding and iron deficiency. In fact, cow's milk is not recommended for infants under six months of age.

In addition, most human adults cannot digest milk. This incapacity is called *lactose intolerance.* I'm sure that you have heard of it; maybe you even suffer from it. In order to digest lactose—the carbohydrate sugar in milk— our bodies require *lactase.* This enzyme is usually present at birth, but, in most humans, its concentration declines with age. As a result, many adults become lactose intolerant and suffer from a number of symptoms after consuming milk or milk products. These symptoms may include bloating, gas, abdominal cramps, nausea, and/or watery stools. Approximately 70 percent of the world's population is lactose intolerant. Lactase deficiency affects 90 percent of Asians, as well as 75 percent of American Blacks and Native Americans. There is also a very high incidence of lactase deficiency in people from the Mediterranean area.

EGG-XAGGERATED BENEFITS

Most of us have been taught that eggs are the perfect protein food, that they contain all of the right amino acids in the right amounts. The protein found in eggs is referred to as *high biological value protein.* As a matter of fact, it was the standard by which all other proteins were once measured. But that has changed. Soy, a plant protein, actually deserves the blue ribbon. Soy is not only a complete protein containing all of the essential amino acids in a practical portion size, but it is also low in saturated fat, high in fiber, and contains no cholesterol. Furthermore, soy contains iron and calcium, "good fats," and *isoflavones*—plant chemicals that have been found to promote a healthy cholesterol profile and to decrease the risk of heart disease, among other potential benefits.

Eggs are way behind when it comes to running in the "heart healthy" race. It is important to realize that one egg contains 213 milligrams of cholesterol, which covers 71 percent (or two-thirds) of the daily recommendations for cholesterol given by the American Dietetic Association, the

American Diabetes Association, the American Heart Association, and the National Cholesterol Education Program. Presently, eggs are considered one of the primary contributors to the development of heart disease.

THE COSTS THAT OUTWEIGH THE BENEFITS

You might say, "Though most adult humans cannot digest milk, *LactAid* and other specialized products can take care of the problem. After all, milk and eggs add variety to the diet, while providing needed calcium and/or protein. So why throw the baby out with the bath water?" Well, a lot of vegan foods are equally nutritious sources of protein and calcium, and they do not carry such high price tags. The regular consumption of milk, milk products (especially whole-fat products), and eggs can result in severe health problems.

Dairy products and eggs are two of the three main culprits causing atherosclerosis (plaques along the walls of the arteries), heart attacks, and strokes. (Meat is the third culprit.) Why? Simply because of their high-fat contents. In *May All Be Fed: Diet for a New World,* John Robbins reports that Finland has the highest incidence of death from heart disease. It also has one of the highest consumption rates of milk and milk products. As a matter of fact, the Finnish eat one and a half times the milk and dairy products that Americans eat each day, and they are one and a half times more likely to die from heart disease than Americans.

When researchers look at the cholesterol and fat levels in vegans, lactovegetarians, lacto-ovovegetarians, and meat-eaters, they find that vegans have the lowest and the most desirable levels. They also have the lowest incidence of death from heart disease. Chapter 12 will explore diet and heart disease in detail.

The Surgeon General's *Report on Nutrition and Health* and the *Healthy People 2000 Objectives* recommend a diet that fulfills the following profile: high in complex carbohydrates; high in dietary fiber; low in total fat, especially saturated fat (the kind found in both milk and eggs); and low in cholesterol, which is found only in foods of animal origin. They also encourage the maintenance of a healthy body weight. These suggestions can easily be followed by committing to veganism. The vegan diet certainly meets the standards for being a heart-healthy diet.

What about all of the low-fat dairy products like skim milk, low-fat yogurt, and low-fat cheese? Unfortunately, "low fat" does not mean decreased risk of obtaining a foodborne illness from these foods. That's a frightening issue unto itself and is discussed next. So, when it comes to eating dairy and egg products, there are more costs than benefits.

THE FACTS ON FOODBORNE ILLNESSES

None of us want to be bothered with worrying whether or not the food in our favorite grocery store is safe. Furthermore, even if we did worry about it, chances are we couldn't pick out the contaminated foods from the uncontaminated ones. Yet food safety is a growing concern, as the reports about food recalls, foodborne illnesses, and resulting deaths increase in frequency.

Every year, foodborne illnesses cause 9,000 deaths and sicken approximately 80 million people. The resulting national cost runs anywhere from $5.6 billion to more than $22 billion per year. And foodborne illnesses are an increasing problem. Most are caused by the consumption of meat, poultry, eggs, milk, and dairy foods that are contaminated with dangerous bacteria.

The November 1997 issue of *U.S. News and World Report* includes an article titled, "O Is for Outbreak." It studies data from the United States Department of Agriculture (USDA) and concludes that meat and poultry products are the source of about 70 percent of foodborne-illness outbreaks. And if you are unlucky enough to become infected with a drug-resistant bacteria, the antibiotics that your doctor prescribes will not help you to get well.

Symptoms and Treatment of Food Poisoning

Usually, the first signs of both *Salmonella* and *E. coli* poisoning are flu-like symptoms. During *Salmonella* poisoning, nausea, crampy abdominal pain, followed by diarrhea, fever, and sometimes vomiting, can occur twelve to forty-eight hours after ingestion of a contaminated food. Stools are often watery, but mucus or blood in the feces is rarely present. These symptoms can persist for one to four days.

Generally, additional fluids and a bland diet is sufficient for treating *Salmonella* poisoning. However, seniors, nursing-home residents, infants, and individuals with HIV (human immunodeficiency virus) or AIDS (acquired immune deficiency syndrome) should be treated with antibiotics. Therefore, consulting with a physician in such cases is necessary.

E. coli is more dangerous than *Salmonella*. It causes severe abdominal cramps and watery diarrhea that can become bloody within the first twenty-four hours of infection. Fever is usually absent or low grade, but there have been rare cases in which fever has reached up to 102.2°F (39°C). The diarrhea can last anywhere from one to eight days in *uncomplicated* infections. For cases that remain uncomplicated, additional fluids and a bland diet should adequately resolve the diarrhea and vomiting. However, some *E. coli* infections get much worse.

About 5 percent of *E. coli* cases become complicated by hemolytic-uremic syndrome (HUS), in which anemia caused by the destruction of red blood cells occurs, as well as acute renal (kidney) failure. The kidney complications are usually sudden but temporary, if treated properly. Thrombotic thrombocytopenic purpura (TTP) is another complication that can occur. TTP can cause HUS, fever, and neurological deficits. Both TTP and HUS develop in the second week of the illness. Individuals who suffer from them usually require admission to a hospital's intensive care unit and then dialysis—a procedure that removes wastes and excess water from the body. Both of these diseases can be fatal, especially if not treated appropriately.

If serious foodborne illness is suspected, you should:

- Call your doctor immediately and seek treatment.

- Wrap and label suspected food and keep it refrigerated for possible inspection by health authorities.

- Notify the Health Hazard Evaluation Board of the Food and Drug Administration's (FDA's) Bureau of Foods.

According to West and Wood's *Foodservice in Institutions,* the U.S. Public Health Service defines a potentially hazardous food as, "Any food which consists in whole or in part of milk or milk products, eggs, meat, poultry, fish, shellfish, edible crustacea, or other ingredients, including synthetic ingredients, in a form capable of supporting rapid and progressive growth of infectious or toxigenic microorganisms." The primary organisms known to cause foodborne illnesses are *Salmonella*; pathogenic *Escherichia coli (E. coli)*; *Vibrio paraehaemolyticus*; and *Compylobacter jejuni*. *Salmonella* and *E. coli* are the two most prevalent microorganisms.

The most commonly reported foods contaminated with *Salmonella* include: dairy products; custards; meats; raw milk; and egg products. Contamination can occur in many ways. Infected cows and chickens, as well as humans with contaminated hands, easily spread this harmful organism. *E. coli* is found in the feces of animals and humans, ultimately making water and soil a possible medium of contamination.

What's in the Milk?

Safe Food: Eating Wisely in a Risky World by Jacobson, Lefferts, and Garland tells us that the use of milk and milk products has been associated with some of the largest food-poisoning outbreaks in the United States. In 1982, approximately 17,000 people in Tennessee became ill after drinking pasteurized milk contaminated with the *Yersinia enterocolitica* bacteria. Pasteurized milk was again the culprit in 1985, when 16,000 people were confirmed as—and as many as 200,000 more suspected of—having been food poisoned by an antibiotic-resistant strain of *Salmonella*. Some of these people died.

Additional instances of large-scale food poisoning have hit the news. Also in 1985, forty-seven fatalities in Southern California resulted from the ingestion of a Mexican-style soft cheese contaminated with *listeria*, another bacteria. This was the largest number of fatalities from food poisoning in recent United States history. (*Listeria* is also highly dangerous, even fatal, to unborn children. Pregnant women are advised to abstain from eating soft cheeses as a preventive measure.) And in 1994, over 224,000 people were sickened by *Salmonella*-contaminated Schwan's ice cream, according to the Centers for Disease Control and Prevention.

What's in the Eggs?

Now for the eggs. One out of every 10,000 eggs is contaminated with *Salmonella*. Most Americans eat over 200 eggs a year, which gives them a pretty good chance, throughout their lifetime, of eating one that is contaminated with this bacteria. From 1985 to 1988, Grade A eggs were responsible for 140 outbreaks of *Salmonella enteriditis*, affecting about 5,000 people and sending 896 of them to the hospital. Furthermore, researchers at the University of Wisconsin found that out of 2,300 laying hens from three flocks, only eight were not infected with *Compylobacter*. Yet most Americans never give a second thought to the possible health hazards of certain foods. They live as if foodborne illness and the bacteria that causes it could never exist in their everyday foods.

In September of 1996, television's *Dateline* reported, ". . . Even an act of Congress hasn't been enough to protect you and your family from a health threat that can hide in foods we all eat. It's a dangerous new strain of an old bacteria—one that is now estimated to sicken and kill even more Americans than *E. coli* in hamburgers. . . ." According to *Dateline,* this contaminant started poisoning people about a decade prior. In 1987, over 400 patients in a New York hospital became sick, and eleven of them died. Three years later, at a convention in Chicago, another 400 people got sick. In Nebraska, a man died after eating homemade ice cream. Then a Pennsylvania woman perished after enjoying a piece of custard pie. And in all of these cases, eggs were the culprit.

The new strain of bacteria in eggs was found and identified as *Salmonella enteriditis (SE)*. This bacteria gets into the eggs even before they are laid. Researchers at the Centers for Disease Control (CDC) believe that *SE* resides in the reproductive tract of the chickens. Unfortunately, infected eggs do not look, taste, or smell differently than uncontaminated eggs.

Researchers found a solution; at around 40°F, the growth of the *SE* bacteria can be contained to safe levels. Now, it was up to the government to make and enforce a law mandating that eggs be kept at a temperature below 45°F immediately after processing. In 1991, Congress passed such a law. It was supported by the egg industry and signed by President George Bush. Yet in southern California, the biggest egg-producing region in the nation, more and more people were being poisoned by *SE*. The problem? Eggs were not being held at the appropriate temperature.

You may think, "That's illegal!" And you're right. However, when Congress passed the law, they failed to do something equally important— they failed to set up a regulatory standard to enforce the law. As a result, at markets across the nation, eggs continued—and continue—to be kept either completely unrefrigerated or refrigerated at inappropriate temperatures for days. And what does the government plan to do at this point? Nothing.

An Important Note of Caution

Though foodborne bacteria most often reside in meat, eggs, and dairy items, any type of food that is not handled properly can become infected. Recently, fruits and vegetables have been the source of several serious food-poisoning outbreaks. According to Luise Light, editor of *The Vegetarian Times*, these outbreaks are due to cross-contamination, which occurs when clean food surfaces, water, and/or people's hands come into contact with bacteria-containing food or soil. That food or soil was previously contaminated when it came into contact with infected meat or the manure of infected livestock.

Understanding Normal & Clinical Nutrition (Third Edition) by Whitney, Cataldo, and Rolfes offers several suggestions on how to avoid consuming contaminants. For starters, be sure to wash your fresh produce in water. Use a scrub brush and rinse it thoroughly. Also, when you want to peel a fruit such as an orange or a grapefruit, do not bite into the skin; use a knife instead. Peel off and discard the outer layers of leafy vegetables such as lettuce. In addition, peel waxed vegetables and fruits. Cucumbers and apples are examples of commonly waxed produce items.

Surface level contaminants are not the only problem. There are also poisons that can grow on foods such as grains and nuts. Moldy foods can present a health risk to humans; mycotoxins are poisons that are produced by molds. *Aflatoxin* is a common mycotoxin and has been found to be carcinogenic (cancer-causing) in experimental animals. It can also be carcinogenic in humans when consumed in unsafe levels over an extended period of time. Cereal grains, nuts (especially peanuts), nutbutters, corn products, and seeds can become contaminated by aflatoxins.

So far, deadly aflatoxin epidemics have occurred only in animals that were fed the contaminated products. However, in 1987 to 1988, thousands of pounds of milk had to be destroyed due to aflatoxin contamination. The mycotoxin got into the milk via the cows who ate contaminated meal.

There are several steps you can take to prevent yourself from consuming unsafe levels of aflatoxin in your food. First, inspect nuts before you eat them. If they appear shriveled, moldy, discolored, or rotten, or if they taste bad, spit them out and throw the food away. Second, do not use moldy grain. Third, refrigerate your nuts and other susceptible foods, especially if you are not planning on using them within a reasonable amount of time. Refrigeration can prevent and minimize the development of aflatoxins.

You can also call the manufacturer of the product you purchase, to see if the company tests for aflatoxin levels. (It is preferable that aflatoxin levels be less than 1 parts per billion.) Arrowhead Mills and Walnut Acres are two examples of natural food manufacturers who regularly test their products for unsafe levels of aflatoxins.

Even the egg industry cannot understand why Congress is not taking more action. Despite the fact that *SE* is now responsible for over 200 deaths and 500,000 illnesses per year, the government of the United States will not enforce its law. Thus, eggs that receive the Department of Agriculture's Grade A stamp of approval, or any other eggs for that matter, could very well contain SE. Forty-five percent of the chicken flocks tested in 1995 registered as positive for SE. No wonder the problem is growing! Presently, one out of every forty Americans will be exposed to SE through eggs.

THE DANGER OF DRUGS AND OTHER CHEMICALS IN YOUR FOOD

It's not just illness-provoking bacteria about which we have to worry when it comes to harmful substances found in milk and eggs. The cows that give us milk and, later, end up on our plates are often given profuse amounts of chemical substances.

Veterinary Drugs

In her book titled *Poisons In Your Plate,* Ruth Winter reveals that there are 750 approved drug products that are used in food animals. These substances include antibiotics (such as penicillin), fertility drugs, pesticides, and hormones. All of these drugs, including some that the FDA has not approved for use on dairy cows, are available without prescription in local farm-feed stores.

What we eat is what we get. The cows are pumped up with drugs. Then we drink their chemical-containing milk and eat their drug-contaminated flesh. Several drugs used in dairy cattle are capable, even at low levels, of causing allergic reactions in a small fraction of milk drinkers. In general, milk is the most common cause of food allergy, and it is conceivable that, in some cases, the offending substance may not be the milk but traces of drugs. Also, some of the veterinary drugs used on food animals are suspected to slightly increase the risk of cancer in humans.

Pesticides

Pesticides such as PCB, DDE, and DDT are terribly harmful. These substances are known as *organochlorines,* and they permeate our food supply. Research on these toxins shows that they, too, may increase cancer risk. Most foods are treated with these substances, and the concentration increases as we move higher on the food chain. Meat, milk, and eggs are the foods that contain the highest doses of organochlorines.

The compounds that make the organochlorines are fat soluble; once they enter the body, they are absorbed into the fat tissue. Animals that are exposed to these toxins retain them in their fat tissues, and their milk is contaminated because milk contains fat. Of course, the flesh also contains organochlorines. People who eat meat and eggs and who drink milk are receiving larger doses of the poisons than people—namely vegans—who avoid these foods.

Women, in particular, are susceptible to the effects of organochlorines, since the breasts are composed almost entirely of fat. Research over the past twenty years has shown that breast tumors in women contain larger amounts of organochlorines than the tissue surrounding the breasts. Organochlorines can also cause excesses of estrogen in the body. Excesses of estrogen clearly have been identified as promoting breast tumors.

From the 1950s to the mid-1970s, the female population in Israel had been experiencing a steady increase in deaths from breast cancer. Then, between 1976 and 1986, there was an unexpected 8-percent drop in this death rate. What happened? In 1978, Israel banned three organochlorine pesticides that previously had been used in cowsheds. This information is highly convincing that chemical pesticides have a direct and detrimental effect on our health.

ABOUT THE ANIMALS

We are not the only ones harmed by the dairy and egg industries. The treatment of the animals that provide these foods is anything but ideal. Cows and chickens are manipulated and mistreated.

The Dairy Industry

Don't forget about poor old Bessie the cow. Imagine just how much milk is consumed every day in the United States alone. Now try to imagine how much milk must be produced to keep up with such a demand. The amazing thing is that the number of dairy cows in the United States has dropped, while milk production continues to soar.

In 1950, 22 million cows were responsible for producing 117 billion pounds of milk. By late 1993, 10 million cows were responsible for supplying 151 billion pounds of milk. How do we get more milk from fewer cows? In 1994, the Food and Drug Administration (FDA) approved the use of *bovine growth hormone (BGT)* and its synthetic version called *recombinant bovine somatotropin (BST)*. BGT is natural to cows, but it can be produced artificially through biotechnology. When BGT or BST is given to cattle through injection, it increases their milk production by 25 percent. As a result, overproduction of milk has become such a problem in the United States that the government has to buy milk in the form of butter and cheese, as well as non-fat dried milk, just to maintain orderly market prices.

The FDA clearly states that these growth hormones are safe for both humans and the cows. However, not everyone feels so positively about it. The approval of BST has met a lot of resistance, and it should. There are reports that the drug can stress cows and make them more susceptible to illness, which harms the cows and the people who eat the food that comes from these cows. Also, there is evidence that BST increases the levels of insulin-like growth factor in milk, which can cause abnormal spleen growth rate as well as tumors in the animals, and increases that risk for certain cancers in humans. While none of these reports have been confirmed, we can surely deduce that the approval of BST demonstrates a belief that we can treat other species as we please, even to the point of an unnatural existence.

The Egg Industry

The egg and poultry industry is not any kinder than the beef and dairy industry. Chickens are treated no better than their milk-producing friends. They get placed into cramped and overcrowded pens that actually make them go crazy. In order to keep the chickens from killing each other in panic and rage, their beaks are snapped off. Then they are subjected to confinement under lights, to promote egg-laying. Finally, when those days are over, they are sent to people like Mr. Perdue and become the chicken on your plate.

It's time to moooove on. The decision is up to you. Are eggs and milk absolute necessities for life and health? Are you able to obtain the necessary nutrients for health maintenance, such as adequate protein and calcium, from vegetarian foods like soy? Do eggs and milk offer the same health benefits as soy and other vegan foods? And finally, can eggs and milk place you at an even greater health risk? It shouldn't take you long to come to the conclusion that you will be doing yourself and the cows and chickens of this world a whole lot of good by turning to a completely plant-based diet.

Part Two

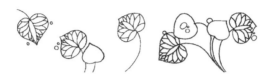

Nutrition
& Vegetarianism
Throughout the Life Cycle

*Knowledge is only beneficial if
it is wisely incorporated into everyday life.*

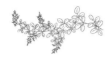 Chapter 4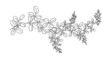

Basic Balancing of the Five Food Groups

Donna Campovich is a 35-year-old divorced mother of two whose family practices veganism. Donna used to feel a twinge of guilt every time she served cornflakes, white-flour biscuits, or white rice. She knew that whole grain products would be healthier, but whose kids will eat them? Then, a little help from a vegetarian magazine changed her family's entire diet. Donna learned some fantastic ways to incorporate more whole grains into her family's meals.

She now makes more oatmeal for breakfast, substitutes some of the white flour with whole wheat flour when she bakes, and mixes her brown rice with spicy tofu. And once Donna made a commitment to become more conscientious about grains, she began to pay better attention to all of the food groups. Now Donna is much more aware of nutritional balance in her family's diet, and she has confidence that it can be achieved without sacrificing taste or variety.

Following a vegetarian diet means more than just going meatless, and following a vegan diet involves more than abstaining from all animal products. A well-planned variety of wholesome and nutritious foods is necessary. The vegan diet should be composed of five food groups: grains, fruits, vegetables, legumes, and nuts/seeds. Vegans must learn as much as they can about these nutrient-dense foods and the necessary amounts of each, in order to achieve a balanced diet. Incidentally, the following information on the five food groups for vegans will contribute to any vegetarian's knowledge of how to maintain a healthy diet.

WHOLE GRAINS

Whole grains are some of the most nutritious foods that we can consume. They are high in protein; complex carbohydrates; fiber; and numerous vitamins and minerals, including iron, calcium, niacin, vitamin B_6, phosphorus, zinc, and thiamin. It is recommended by the Vegetarian Food Pyramid that six to eleven servings of whole grains be consumed daily, in the forms of cereals, breads, and pastas (see Figure 4.1 below.).

There is a difference between the terms *whole grains* and *grains*. Whole grains have been processed only slightly, and thus have not had most or all of their nutrients removed. They contain significantly more nutrients than grains that have been heavily processed and refined. It is true that some processing is necessary to render grains more digestible, but heavy processing and refining strip the foods of their natural health benefits.

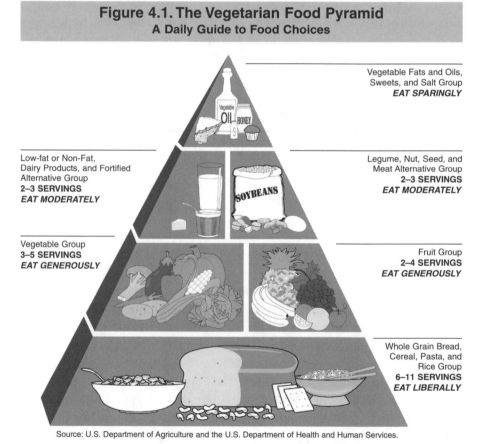

Figure 4.1. The Vegetarian Food Pyramid
A Daily Guide to Food Choices

Vegetable Fats and Oils, Sweets, and Salt Group
EAT SPARINGLY

Low-fat or Non-Fat, Dairy Products, and Fortified Alternative Group
2–3 SERVINGS
EAT MODERATELY

Legume, Nut, Seed, and Meat Alternative Group
2–3 SERVINGS
EAT MODERATELY

Vegetable Group
3–5 SERVINGS
EAT GENEROUSLY

Fruit Group
2–4 SERVINGS
EAT GENEROUSLY

Whole Grain Bread, Cereal, Pasta, and Rice Group
6–11 SERVINGS
EAT LIBERALLY

Source: U.S. Department of Agriculture and the U.S. Department of Health and Human Services.

A study reported in *Tufts University Health & Nutrition Letter* in 1998 followed more than 30,000 females for nine years and found that the women who chose whole grains for at least three of their daily grain servings had a 30-percent less likelihood of heart attack. The healthful contents of whole grains—including fiber; nutrients such as vitamin E and magnesium; phytochemicals; antioxidants; and phytoestrogents (plant hormones) —are believed to play a role in that significant cardiovascular advantage.

All cereal grains contain three vital components. The starchy endosperm comprises about 83 percent of the grain and is rich in protein. The protective outer layer, known as the bran, constitutes only 5 percent of the grain and is rich in the B vitamins and in minerals. The embryo or germ is the third and final component, and makes up only 2 to 3 percent of the grain. It is rich in protein, fat, and minerals.

When grains are processed or milled, the bran and the germ are removed. Most people are unaware of the amount of nutrients that are stripped away with this removal process. That is because we are taught (even by up-to-date nutrition textbooks) that the endosperm contains the majority of necessary nutrients. However, both the bran and the germ contain significant amounts of nutrients not provided by the endosperm alone.

Certain members of the food and health industries pacify our concerns by telling us that the depleted nutrients in processed or milled grains are replaced through a process known as *enrichment*. You probably have noticed that some grain products contain the word *enriched* on the package. This is a good advertising ploy, for the term makes us think that the food items have been enhanced in some manner. But enriched foods are foods that originally have been depleted of their natural nutrients and, in many cases, only a portion of those nutrients are replaced or put back. The process does not make a product nutritionally equal to its natural form.

Simply stated, whole grains are healthier. They provide certain vitamins and minerals that processed and enriched foods do not contain, such as zinc and vitamin B_6. Look at Table 4.1 on page 40, which compares three different types of flours: whole wheat; un-enriched; and enriched. The information is adapted from *Bowes and Church's Food Values of Portions Commonly Used* (Sixteenth Edition) by Jean A.T. Pennington. You will notice that the whole wheat flour is the healthiest, by far.

There is a very important difference between enriched foods and *fortified foods*. The latter are foods to which have been added nutrients that the foods either never contained in the first place or contained in insignificant amounts. Some good examples are: milk with vitamin D; orange juice with calcium; and flour with folacin. Fortification began when the dairy indus-

Table 4.1. Comparing Flours			
	Whole Wheat Flour	**Un-Enriched Flour**	**Enriched Flour**
Protein	23.00 g	11.60 g	12.00 g
Fiber	16.00 g	0.30 g	3.00 g
Calcium	200.00 mg	20.00 mg	17.00 mg
Zinc	4.40 mg	—	0.80 mg

try started fortifying milk with vitamin D because many American children's diets were deficient in that nutrient. Today, more and more products are enhanced with vitamins and minerals. Even several of the cold cereals, such as *Total* and *Product 19*, are heavily fortified. Fortified foods are excellent nutrient sources.

The following tips offer suggestions on how to increase the amount of whole grains in your diet:

•   Eat whole wheat bread, instead of wheat bread or white bread.

•   Add whole grains like barley, couscous, millet, and brown rice to your meals.

•   When baking, use whole wheat pastry flour instead of white flour.

•   Use the "half-n-half method" to slowly introduce whole grains to your family—that is, serve half white rice and half brown rice on each plate; use half white flour and half whole wheat flour in your baking.

•   Add wheat germ and bran to loaves, cookies, breads, cereals, and other foods.

•   Purchase a whole grains cookbook and try out some new dishes.

FRUITS AND VEGETABLES

Fruits and vegetables provide tremendous variety, color, and flavor to the vegetarian diet. They also play a major role in the prevention of many chronic diseases, including cancer and heart disease. The foods in these two groups are good sources of vitamin C; beta-carotene; vitamin K; potassium; and fiber.

According to an article in the November 24, 1997 edition of *U.S. News and World Report,* Americans have increased their fruit and vegetable consumption by 70 percent since 1950. This is partially due to the increase in the number of recommended servings per day. In 1993, the Four Food Group Plan was replaced by the Food Guide Pyramid. The old food plan recommended four servings of fruits and vegetables, while the Food Guide Pyramid recommends five to nine servings per day.

Fruits and vegetables provide numerous health benefits. Many are discussed in Part Three of this book, in regards to the prevention of specific diseases. For example, these two food groups are excellent sources of antioxidants, which have documented roles in cancer prevention. Among the antioxidants are beta-carotene and vitamin C. Several studies have shown that low intakes of fruits and vegetables that are rich in beta-carotene and vitamin C result in higher incidences of cancer, especially colon and stomach cancer. (Generally, vegetables and fruits that are orange-yellow in color are rich in beta-carotene.) Be sure to make antioxidant-rich fruits and vegetables part of your daily diet. For more information on diet and cancer, see Chapter 15.

You have countless options when it comes to nourishing yourself on fruits and vegetables. For example, in addition to fresh fruits, dried fruits are convenient and tasty treats that provide calcium and considerable amounts of iron. For more information, see Table A.2: Calcium-Rich Foods on pages 236 to 237, and "Table A.5: Iron-Rich Foods on pages 240 to 241.

Also, fruit and vegetable juices are delicious sources of vitamins and minerals. In *The Complete Juicer,* author Lionel Martinez states, "Drinking three to four glasses of fruit and vegetable juices at different times during the day is an excellent way to insure a continuous daily supply of nutrients." I personally enjoy childhood memories of making juice with my siblings and my mom. We were delighted with the colored liquids that the fruits and vegetables yielded. Combining textures and flavors can be quite an exercise in art. So have fun while you get healthy; buy yourself a juicer and start creating!

Keep in mind that your servings of vegetables should include at least two different types: dark green, leafy vegetables and cruciferous vegetables. Dark green, leafy vegetables, such as spinach, collard greens, kale, mustard greens, and broccoli, are excellent sources of beta-carotene, vitamin C, calcium, and iron. Cruciferous vegetables, such as cabbage, cauliflower, broccoli, Brussels sprouts, turnips, and rutabagas, contain indoles, dithiolthiones, and other chemical compounds that are essential for the destruction of carcinogens (cancer-causing agents).

LEGUMES (ESPECIALLY SOYBEANS)

Legumes, commonly known as beans, come in a variety of shapes, sizes, and colors—from the green and orange split peas to the black-eye peas, and from the kidney-shaped lima beans to the disk-shaped lentils. Legumes are an essential part of the vegetarian diet. They provide significant nutrients, including: protein; fiber; iron; calcium; zinc; folacin; and the B-complex vitamins. Plus, it is not only nutrition that pushes beans to the forefront, but also the fact that they are inexpensive. By all means, beans should be the vegetarian's "meat." The vegan should eat at least one to three servings of legumes per day.

Soybeans are among the most popular, praised, and researched legumes. For years, researchers and health professionals believed that no vegetable protein was equal to meat protein. But modern research has proven that soybeans and soy products are excellent sources of protein, fiber, and many vitamins and minerals. Soybeans contain all nine essential amino acids; soy is a complete protein. In fact, soy protein is preferable to meat protein because it is lower in fat, has no cholesterol, and contains complex carbohydrates and fiber.

The advantages of including soy in your diet are numerous. Studies have shown that it is instrumental in the reduction of blood-cholesterol levels and, thus, its consumption is associated with a decreased risk of heart disease. Research is also finding a connection between soy and reduced risk of cancer and osteoporosis. Soy is also being researched for its potential in relieving certain menopausal symptoms.

Incorporating soy into your diet may not be as difficult as you might think. Current food technology has developed an exquisite variety of products made from soy that are readily available at your nearest health food store, and even at your local grocery store. Consider the following soy-foods, which are only a few of the many: miso; soy cheese; soy flour; soy protein isolate; soy yogurt; soybean oil; tempeh; and tofu (see "Tofu Talk" on page 43).

NUTS AND SEEDS

Nuts and seeds are probably the least popular of the vegetarian foods. That is a pity, especially since they are rich in a number of vitamins and minerals in which the vegetarian (especially vegan) diet is otherwise often low. For example, take the mineral zinc, which Chapter 5 discusses in detail. Most of

Tofu Talk

Tofu is definitely the most popular soyfood, as it is the most readily available and the most publicized. For centuries, tofu has been the staple protein for millions of people throughout Asia. It is made by coagulating soymilk with calcium or magnesium salt (making it an excellent source of calcium when calcium salts are used). Then the whey is squeezed out and what we know as tofu is left.

There are many types of tofu. Most varieties have very smooth textures and high moisture content, though some are crumbly and somewhat dry. Tofu is rather bland; it does not have a strong taste on its own. This makes it extremely versatile; you can season it to make it taste like whatever you desire. Tofu is used as the base for soy mayonnaise, salad dressings, dips, and puddings. It is used in place of egg in egg salad and to substitute for cheese on pizza. Tofu can be baked, fried, sautéed, scrambled, and even grilled.

There have been recent complaints that tofu is high in fat. Like other plant foods, it does contain fat. That's okay—we need some fat in our diets, and it's much better to get this fat from a healthful substance that contains disease-inhibiting components. The bottom line is that tofu causes less health problems than meat. In nations in which diets are predominantly meat-based, including the United States, heart disease rates are sky-high. Quite differently, in Asia, where meat consumption is low and tofu/soy consumption is high, the people do not suffer and die from heart disease to the same alarming extent.

the nutrition articles that argue against vegetarianism claim zinc is found primarily in animal foods. Thus, literature on nutrition often claims that vegetarians are at a higher risk of zinc deficiency. But nuts and seeds are excellent sources of zinc—and iron too! You may be thinking, "Yeah, but they're also high in fat." That's true, but nuts and seeds contain mostly good fats.

When it comes to fats, plant foods hold several advantages over animal products. First, plants contain more poly- and monounsaturated fats, and less saturated fat, with the exception of coconut and palm-kernel oils. Both poly- and monounsaturated fats actually play a role in the *prevention* of heart disease. Saturated fat, on the other hand, is well-known for its role in *causing* heart disease.

Beverages and Dietary Balancing

Most people do not give a second thought to the role beverages play in daily nutrition. But beverages are easier to consume than food, and the nutrients they provide can get into our bloodstream more quickly. This is due to the fact that, for the most part, beverages do not require additional digestion.

Unfortunately, America's favorite beverages are caffeinated. According to the National Coffee Association's annual survey, 49 percent of Americans consume coffee. The average annual consumption for adults is 26.7 gallons, or over 400 cups. We tend to overlook the fact that caffeine is officially classified as an addictive drug, just like nicotine and heroin. It is also a depressant; caffeine gives you a temporary high, and then brings you down lower than you previously were, causing you to yearn for an additional high. And so the cycle begins again.

Use your beverages to contribute to your nutrition, and start with water. Fifty-five to sixty percent of an adult's body weight is water, making it the most abundant and essential nutrient in the body. We can survive weeks without food, but we can only survive a few days without water. An inadequate intake of water can lead to dehydration, which eventually causes a number of life-threatening electrolyte imbalances, as well as other conditions such as constipation. Adults should drink at least 8 cups of water every day.

Fruit and vegetable juices certainly should be included in your diet. Fruit juices, such as apple juice, orange juice, and grape juice, are good sources of vitamin C. Vegetable juices made from carrots, celery, and beets provide vitamin A and other important nutrients.

Herbal teas are becoming more popular. If used appropriately, they can greatly enhance your diet. Peppermint and spearmint teas make delicious, caffeine-free hot or cold drinks. They are known to aid the digestion process and have been used to relieve nausea and cold symptoms for centuries. Chamomile tea is widely recognized for its soothing effect; some people drink a cup in the evening to relax. Chamomile also seems to aid digestion, and it has been known to relieve various head, skeletal, and muscular aches and pains. As is evident through these brief descriptions, herbal teas have medicinal values. Please realize that there are cautions to be taken with the potent leaves that make tea. It is best to seek the advice of a health professional with a background in herbs before you begin trying different varieties of herbal teas. For more information on the ways that teas can positively affect your health, read *Healing Teas* by Marie Nadine Antol.

Postum and roma are two options for those who desire something similar to coffee, or for anyone who simply would like a warm drink on a wintery night. They are both caffeine free, yet they provide a coffee-like flavor, color, and aroma. Postum is made from a special blend of rich, roasted grains, including bran and wheat. Roma is made from roasted malt, roasted barley, and roasted chicory, and has a stronger flavor that is closer to coffee. Both roma and postum are very low in calories. Of course, if you add non-dairy creamers, soymilk, sugar, and/or molasses, the calorie count will increase.

Our beverage decisions directly affect our daily nutrition. Those decisions can either harm or help us. It may take a little practice and some significant habit-breaking, but in the long run, drinking healthy beverages can make a big difference.

The second advantage of consuming fat-containing plant foods over fat-containing animal products is that many of the plant foods also provide significant amounts of fiber and complex carbohydrates. Fibrous foods are associated with such benefits as enhanced cardiovascular and digestive health and cancer prevention. (See "The Benefits of a High-Fiber Vegan Diet," page 173.) And quite simply, we need carbohydrates, including complex carbohydrates, for energy.

Finally, there is no cholesterol in plant foods, but plenty of cholesterol in animal products. That 3-ounce serving of broiled steak contains 86 milligrams of cholesterol, while the nuts and seeds have none. So even though nuts and seeds are technically high in fats, they can contribute to your health in many ways.

It is too easy to meet and exceed the daily requirements for fat by topping our baked potatoes, vegetables, and practically every other food with products such as margarine, butter, mayonnaise, and cheese. Instead of depending on these unhealthy items, which are high in saturated fats, consider obtaining most of your fat from nuts and seeds. Try nutbutters on your toast or bagels. A serving of cashew butter, for example, will provide more protein, carbohydrates, calcium, iron, magnesium, phosphorus, and zinc than a serving of margarine, plus the nutbutter will provide fiber and contains less fat. Whatever you do, do not use both nutbutters and margarine (or other "fat" spreads). Nuts are to be used as a *substitute* for other fats. Eating nuts while maintaining your previous intake of fat most likely will result in undesirable fat and calorie intake.

It is important to realize that nuts have been recognized as foods that prevent chronic disease. In 1993, the *New England Journal of Medicine* published an article on the effects of walnuts on cholesterol levels. The subjects were separated into two groups of men. Both groups were placed on cholesterol-lowering diets which were similar in their total fat, protein, carbohydrate, and fiber contents. One group received walnuts as a substitute for other fatty foods like potato chips, margarine, butter, and meat. The walnut diet contained more polyunsaturated fatty acids than the non-walnut group. While the cholesterol levels of the individuals in both groups went down in response to the low-cholesterol diets, the subjects in the walnut group exhibited an additional 10-percent decrease in serum-cholesterol levels.

In 1992, Fraser and colleagues published a study that was performed on a number of California Seventh-day Adventists and showed that a moderate nut consumption is associated with a reduction in the risk of heart attacks and death from heart disease. More studies need to be done with a variety of different subjects before we can come to a solid conclusion, but nuts seem to have a protective effect against cardiovascular disease.

Nuts and seeds do have an important place in the vegetarian diet, and in every diet, though they should be eaten moderately due to their fat content. The vegetarian should consume at least one serving of nuts and seeds—that is, 1 ounce of whole/ground nuts or 1 tablespoon of nutbutter—daily. When snacking, eat raw or dry roasted nuts, as opposed to those that have been roasted in oils.

DAILY VEGAN FOOD PATTERN

To be a healthy vegan, you must make sure that you eat a variety of foods from the five vegan food groups. You will note, however, that the food pattern in Table 4.2 on page 47 lists the amount of daily servings suggested for seven food groups. Since soy provides so many benefits to health and nutrition, it has been made into a food group. Also, vitamin B_{12}- and D-fortified foods have been made into a group. Include your fortified food serving in the food group under which it falls. For example, *Whole Grain Total*—a fortified product—should be counted under the whole grain group, while it also meets the fortified food group.

Table 4.2. Daily Food Pattern for the Vegan Female		
Food Group	**Serving Size**	**Servings/Day**
Whole grain products (bread; cereal; rice; pasta)	1 slice; ½ bagel; ½ cup	6–11
Fruits; fruit juices	1 medium piece; ½ cup chopped; ¼ cup dried; 6 oz	2–5
Vegetables; vegetable juice; dark green, leafy vegetables	½ cup cooked; 1 cup raw; 4 oz	2–4 1–3
Tofu; meat analogs; soymilk/soy beverages; other protein-rich soy products	4 oz	2–4
Legumes/beans	½ cup	1–3
Nuts and seeds (including nutbutters)	1 oz; 2 tablespoons	1–2
Vitamin B$_{12}$ and vitamin D-fortified foods (for example, soymilk; dry cereals)	As specified for the food group.	1–2

The pattern in Table 4.2 is designed for vegan females in each stage of life, from adolescence to pregnancy to the senior years. Choosing foods from each of the food groups will ensure an adequate intake of essential nutrients. If your protein and calorie needs are closer to 40 to 50 grams of protein and 1,800 calories per day, focus on the lower half of the ranges. If you require more protein and calories, focus on the higher ranges. Adjustments should be made where appropriate with the advice of a nutrition

Table 4.3. Sample Menu

Breakfast	*Lunch*	*Dinner*
2 whole wheat pancakes with syrup/molasses	1 whole wheat pita pocket filled with ½ cup seasoned tofu	1 cup vegan lasagne
2 vegan sausages	½ cup salad for pita	1½ cups spinach/ broccoli/chickpea salad
1 cup fruit salad sprinkled with ground nuts	1 orange or 1 kiwi	2 tablespoons salad dressing
8 oz *EdenSoy Extra* (soymilk beverage)	6 oz soy yogurt	½ cup butternut squash
4 oz calcium-fortified orange juice	4 oz *V-8* drink	1 whole wheat roll
		2 oatmeal cookies
		8 oz apricot nectar

professional. To record your personal food pattern goals, use the chart provided in Appendix D, page 255.

Though the pattern in Table 4.2 is designed for the vegan female, vegetarians who include milk, dairy products, and/or eggs can also design their diets around this pattern. Milk, dairy foods, and eggs would be incorporated into the tofu and other soyfoods category. Be sure to limit egg yolks to no more than three per week, and to consume low-fat dairy products.

Table 4.3 provides a menu for three balanced meals in accordance with the daily meal pattern given on page 47. It offers a delicious combination of flavors and textures, and the food choices will leave you feeling wonderfully alive.

It is only through learning about our bodies and the nutrients that are necessary to sustain life that we will be able to make sound and reasonable decisions on how to balance nutrition. This chapter has discussed the five basic food groups for vegans, and has explained the amounts of each that should be consumed in the daily diet. The next chapter offers in-depth discussions on specific key nutrients—how they help us; how much we need; from where we can get them. Vegetarianism is not just about *avoiding* certain foods; it's also about *choosing* foods rich in nutrients.

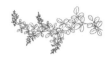 # Chapter 5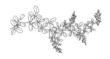

The Deal
on Deficiencies

Upon graduating from college, Melissa Ronan, a lifetime vegetarian and a vegan for the past four years, decided to give six months of volunteer service. She signed up for a program that worked on developing housing and teaching English in a small African community. Before she could begin her assignment, Melissa was asked to undergo several health exams, including a blood profile to investigate nutritional status. Melissa was a little concerned; since she made the switch to veganism, many people insisted that Melissa's diet was surely lacking in certain vitamins and minerals. But when the results of her labwork came back, Melissa was all smiles. The medical staff explained that Melissa was wonderfully healthy—whatever she was doing was working just fine. She now has the evidence she needed to feel confident in veganism.

Many long-time vegetarians, and vegans in particular, have become accustomed to hearing hundreds of opinions about what is missing in their diets. These opinions flow from every direction—from health professionals, family members, coworkers, next door neighbors. "A vegan diet does not contain the high-quality protein that the body needs." "Vitamin B_{12} is not found in plant foods, which proves that we are supposed to eat meat." One nutrition textbook states, "Nutrients that commonly present problems to vegetarians include iron, zinc, calcium, and vitamins B_{12} and D."

What most people do not realize is that these nutrients do not present problems for intelligent vegetarians who eat balanced diets. As a matter of fact, the "vegetarians-are-deficient" advocates should take a closer look at the diet of most meat-eaters, who tend to eat insufficient amounts of the plant foods that are known to decrease the risk of many chronic diseases. The volumes of research show that vegetarians, including vegans, are healthier than most of their meat-eating counterparts, and that deficiencies are rare. The *Journal of the American Dietetic Association* states, "It is the position of the American Dietetic Association (ADA) that appropriately planned vegetarian diets are healthful, are nutritionally adequate, and provide health benefits in the prevention and treatment of certain diseases." The same journal also confirms that vegan and lacto-ovovegetarian diets are suitable for every stage of life. This chapter will discuss what are commonly and often wrongly thought to be deficiencies in the vegetarian/vegan diet.

PROTEIN

Protein is one of the three major nutrients that are essential for healthy growth and muscular development. (The other two are carbohydrates and fats.) It acts as various hormones, which regulate important body functions. Protein helps the body fight infection. Furthermore, it helps maintain the body's fluid and acid-base balance. And, in the form of enzymes, protein aids in the digestion of food. These are just a few of protein's roles.

The Quality of Plant Protein

Many nutrition professionals have long been concerned with adequate protein intake for the vegetarian. However, research has shown that plant proteins are able to support the nutritional needs of human beings. In fact, plant proteins provide 65 percent of the world's supply of protein, predominantly in the form of cereal grains.

Plant proteins are *not* necessarily incomplete proteins, though many people still refer to them as such. Legumes and grains contain all nine essential amino acids. It is true that some plant proteins, when eaten in practical amounts, do not contain enough of a particular amino acid to meet our needs. But that does not pose a problem for the vegetarian, because the consumption of a *combination* of whole grains, legumes, nuts/seeds, and certain fruits and vegetables will supply an adequate intake.

For years, vegetarians across the globe diligently ate rice and beans at the same meal. They faithfully fixed peanut butter and jelly sandwiches for their children. Why? Because they were taught to complement or combine proteins within the same meal. This is not a bad idea, but it is not always necessary. Simply make sure that you meet your total calorie and protein needs for the day within your three meals.

Soy is an example of a complete plant protein and is perfectly capable of being the primary source of protein in a healthy diet. Why did it take so long for scientists to realize the quality of plant proteins, particularly soy proteins? Because the test procedures that were used in the past yielded results that were appropriate for rats, not for humans. The new method that evaluates protein quality without using non-human subjects (called the protein digestibility corrected amino acid score, or PDCAAS) yields a score of 1.0—the highest possible score—for soy protein. This means that soy protein matches the quality of milk protein and egg white protein, and it's actually higher in quality than beef protein, which scores 0.92. The consumption of soy is associated with the prevention and/or treatment of heart disease, cancer, diabetes, kidney disease, osteoporosis, and menopausal symptoms.

Plant proteins have several advantages over animal proteins. They are rich in disease-fighting nutrients such as fiber, and in the case of soy, also rich in isoflavones. Plant proteins contain no cholesterol, and they emphasize mono- and polyunsaturated fats, instead of saturated fat. In addition, many plant proteins are rich sources of both calcium and iron.

SUGGESTED INTAKE AND SOURCES OF PROTEIN

The protein requirement for adults is 0.8 gram/kilogram of body weight. You can easily calculate your protein requirement by dividing your weight in pounds by 2.2 (to get your weight in kilograms), and then by multiplying the answer by 0.8. For example, if you weigh 120 pounds, you would divide 120 by 2.2, yielding 55. Then you would multiply 55 by 0.8, yielding 44. This means you should consume 44 grams of protein per day. Table 5.1 (page 52) provides the already-calculated figures for several different weights.

Some examples of protein-rich plant foods are soy (discussed above) and other legume products, nuts/nutbutters, whole grain cereals and breads, and toasted wheat germ. For specific information on such foods and their protein content, see Appendix A, page 233.

CALCIUM

Calcium is the most abundant mineral in the human body. Ninety-nine percent of it is found in the bones and the teeth. The other one percent is contained in the blood and body fluids. Calcium serves a number of functions. It gives strength and structure to the bones and teeth. It is necessary for muscle contraction and relaxation. This mineral is also involved in the formation of blood clots and is necessary for the transmission of nerve impulses. Calcium helps regulate the transportation of ions into the cells and is critical for the delivery of messages within each cell. Given these major functions, it is easy to understand why maintaining a positive calcium balance is so important.

Table 5.1. Daily Required Protein Intake		
Weight in Pounds	**Weight in Kilograms**	**Protein Requirement in Grams**
100	45	36
110	50	40
120	55	44
130	59	47
140	64	51
150	68	54
160	73	58
170	77	62
180	82	66
190	86	69
200	91	73

Factors That Affect Calcium Levels

The symptoms of calcium deficiency include osteoporosis (bone loss) in adults and stunted growth in children. If you become low in blood calcium, your body starts pulling the calcium from your bones. While the bones contain an abundant supply, they weaken as more and more calcium is taken from them. Thus, they are at greater risk of fracturing and breaking. Knowing the factors that affect calcium balance can help us to maintain an adequate supply in the blood, and therefore allow us to preserve the health of our bones.

Phytate and Oxalic Acid. There has been much debate surrounding the roles of phytate (a particular type of fiber) and oxalic acid—both found in certain fruits and vegetables—in relation to impaired calcium balance. These substances are natural to many foods. While some research has shown that phytate binds to minerals like calcium and prevents them from being absorbed, most researchers conclude that phytate does not affect calcium absorption *significantly*. Thus, we should recognize that phytate does reduce the amount of absorbable calcium in food, but not to the extent that is worrisome.

Oxalic acid, on the other hand, poses a considerable problem. Some foods that appear to be excellent sources of calcium should not be considered as such, due to their high content of oxalic acid. Examples of these foods are: rhubarb; spinach; berries; chocolate; cola beverages; and teas (not herbals). Soybeans also contain a lot of oxalic acid, but they are the one exception to the rule. The body absorbs calcium from soybeans almost as well as it does from milk, even though soybeans contain significant amounts of both phytate and oxalic acid. In fact, a study published in *The Soy Connection* in 1997 examined calcium absorption and found no differences in the amounts of calcium absorbed from tofu (soy curd), cheese, calcium carbonate, and nonfat dry milk.

Due to the phytate and oxalic acid content in some fruits and vegetables, you might think that women who eat high amounts of these foods, such as vegetarian women, have a higher incidence of osteoporosis. It is surprising to learn that vegetarian women have significantly lower incidences of osteoporosis when compared with nonvegetarian women. How is this possible? Well, here's a high point of the *vegan* diet. Some vegetable foods have been found to yield *greater* calcium absorption than milk. These foods include kale greens; broccoli; turnip greens; watercress; rutabaga; radishes; mustard greens; kohlrabi; cauliflower; cabbage; and Brussels sprouts. Vegans tend to eat more of these foods, which gives them an edge when it comes to absorbing calcium.

Protein. Protein's effect on calcium balance has been the subject of ongoing research. Some studies conclude that meat-based, high-protein diets cause a significant loss of calcium in the urine. A study conducted by Johnson and colleagues found that when put on a diet that included 48 grams of protein and 500 milligrams of calcium per day, young people had no net calcium loss. When these subjects' protein intakes were increased to 141 grams per day, they experienced significant amounts of calcium loss in the urine, even though they were also consuming 1,400 milligrams of calcium daily.

The American diet provides excess daily protein due to the consumption of meat, eggs, and dairy products. This increases the calcium demand in the body. People who consume lower amounts of protein per day have lower calcium requirements. The vegetarian diet provides adequate protein without overtaxing the body and requiring calcium amounts that are difficult to maintain. In fact, the American Dietetic Association has concluded that vegan diets have a calcium-sparing effect due to their lower protein and more alkaline-based content.

Phosphorus. Phosphorus *reduces* the loss of calcium from the urine. Vegetarian foods like beans, whole grains, and nuts are excellent sources of phosphorus. Some researchers reported that since meat is also a good source of phosphorus, calcium loss from the high protein content in meat is off-set. However, a study conducted by Hegsted and associates found that increasing dietary protein resulted in significant amounts of urinary calcium loss at both high and low phosphorus intakes. They also found that the high-protein, low-phosphorus diet caused more calcium excretion than the high-protein, high-phosphorus diet.

Sodium. Sodium can work against the body's ability to absorb calcium. It has been found to increase the excretion of calcium in the urine. According to *Modern Nutrition in Health and Disease,* edited by Maurice Shils, the addition of just 3 grams of sodium chloride per day to a regular diet promoted 7.5 percent of a post-menopausal woman's skeletal calcium to be lost over a ten-year period. This alone can increase her risk for osteoporosis. By simply cutting down on your salt intake, you can help your body retain more calcium.

Caffeine. America's favorite beverage ingredient—caffeine—not only increases the urinary excretion of calcium, but also causes an increased secretion of calcium into the gut, where it is expelled through the feces. So in the long run, those caffeinated soft drinks, coffees, and teas heighten addictive cravings while reducing your health.

Vitamin D. When it comes to calcium levels, this is one substance you'll want more of. The presence of vitamin D in your diet will strongly enhance your absorption of calcium. Vitamin D is discussed in greater detail later in this chapter (see page 60).

Suggested Intake and Sources of Calcium

The 19- to 50-year-old vegetarian female should strive to obtain a calcium intake of *at least* 800 to 1,000 milligrams per day from food sources. If you fall into this age bracket, you can obtain this amount of calcium by eating at least two servings of foods that contain 200 milligrams or more of calcium per serving, in addition to well-balanced meals. For a list of calcium-rich vegan foods, see Table A.2 on page 236. A few examples are collard greens, black-eye peas, calcium-set tofu, *Soymage* cheese, and *White Wave Dairyless Yogurt.*

Don't forget to get an adequate amount of vitamin D in your diet as well, as this will aid calcium absorption. Avoid excessive amounts of protein, as well as high intakes of salt and caffeine in your diet. Continue to eat plenty of fruits, vegetables, and whole grains.

The American Dietetic Association (ADA), in their position paper on vegetarian diets, suggests that vegetarians may require less calcium than nonvegetarians because their diets are lower in protein and are more alkaline. The ADA finds that the United States recommendations for calcium intake are really geared toward the individual on the average, meat-based American diet. The association proposes that since vegetarians, according to studies, absorb and retain a greater amount of dietary calcium than meat-eaters, and since calcium deficiency is rare in vegetarians, there is hardly reason to assume that calcium intake that falls below the RDA will cause vegetarians any health problems. But since calcium requirements in vegans have not been individually studied or determined, it would be wise to aim for the amount recommended by the Daily Reference Intake (DRI): 1,000 to 1,300 milligrams.

IRON

Iron is a mineral that serves several critical functions in the body. It allows oxygen to be transported to the tissues in the form of hemoglobin and to be stored in the tissues in the form of myoglobin. Iron is also involved in the transport of electrons. Meat is the main source of iron in the American diet. As a result, intake has become a worrisome issue for many vegetarians. This mineral especially concerns health professionals because iron deficiency is the most common deficiency in humans, affecting over 500 million people throughout the world.

Factors That Affect Iron Levels

Nutrition During Pregnancy, published by National Academy Press, identifies six factors that are associated with a heightened risk of iron deficiency: pregnancy (the second and third trimesters); multiple gestation (pregnancy in which there is more than one fetus); diets low in both meat and ascorbic acid; menorrhagia (loss of more than 80 milliliters of blood per month); blood donation more than three times per year; and chronic use of aspirin. Lack of adequate iron can lead to anemia; see "Iron Deficiency Anemia" on page 56.

It is important to note that there are two forms of iron found in foods. One is called *heme iron* and is found exclusively in animal flesh. The other is *non-heme iron* and is contained in plant foods, as well as in animal flesh. Of the two forms of iron, heme iron is believed to be absorbed more easily by the body. Does this mean that we should eat meat? Of course not. Non-heme iron is not absorbed as easily, but learning how to enhance its absorption will help.

There are several substances and foods that are believed to inhibit iron absorption. These include: phytate (discussed in relation to calcium on page 52); plant polyphenolics (certain plant chemicals); high dietary amounts of zinc and other minerals; soy protein; bran; milk; eggs; tea; coffee; calcium-rich antacids; and calcium phosphates. You are probably thinking that you are bound to be iron deficient because you consume at least half or more of these foods. But before you go on a rampage to eliminate all phytate or soy protein from your diet, we must take a look at the whole picture.

Ascorbic acid, commonly known as vitamin C, can increase the absorption of non-heme iron three to four times! Foods that contain vita-

Iron Deficiency Anemia

Anemia literally means "too little blood" and refers to a condition involving any of the following: too few red blood cells; red blood cells that are immature or too small; red blood cells that contain too little hemoglobin to carry the normal amount of oxygen to the tissues. Anemia is not a disease itself; it is a symptom. Some examples of conditions from which anemia can result are nutrient deficiencies (such as lack of iron, folate, and vitamin B_{12}), excessive bleeding, excessive red blood cell destruction, and defective red blood cell formation.

Iron deficiency refers to the state of being without iron stores. Iron deficiency anemia refers to the condition in which there are small, pale red blood cells resulting from an iron deficiency. If you experience any of the following symptoms, you may suffer from iron deficiency anemia:

- fatigue
- itching
- poor attention span
- poor wound healing

- lowered immunity (general)
- reduced resistance to colds
- reduced physical fitness

Ask your doctor to do a test that will yield your iron levels. It involves a simple blood sample that is then sent to a lab for analysis.

min C—for example, apples, oranges and other citrus fruits, and potatoes—must be eaten with the iron-containing foods in order for them to
have an effect on iron absorption. Vegetarians should not have problems
with this dietary task, as they typically consume plenty of vitamin C-rich
fruits and vegetables.

Now, do vegetarians need to worry about poor iron absorption as a
result of a high phytate intake? Research on this very topic answers this
question, and you may find the results quite encouraging. A study conducted by Brune, Rossander, and Hallberg, published in 1989, included four
men and nine women, all of whom were 35 to 76 years old. The study was
performed with the purpose of determining the long-term effects of a high-
phytate diet on iron absorption. All of the subjects were vegetarians, some
vegans, who had high phytate intake for several years. The researchers
found that the participants had very healthy iron profiles. Another study,
performed by Anderson, Gibson, and Sabry and published in 1981, looked
at the iron status of fifty-six long-term vegetarian women and found that,
despite the inclusion of factors believed to inhibit iron absorption, the
women maintained healthy iron levels.

How are vegetarians able to maintain good iron stores despite their
high phytic intakes? As mentioned above, ascorbic acid (vitamin C) is a
powerful promoter of iron absorption. The vegetarian's typical high intake
of vitamin C, as well as citric, malic, and tartaric acids from fruits and vegetables, is believed to counteract the inhibition of iron absorption that
would otherwise occur with a high-phytate diet. In addition, vegetarians
who exclude tea, coffee, milk, and eggs from their diets have eliminated
additional sources that can inhibit their iron absorption.

Suggested Intake and Sources of Iron

The RDA for iron for adult women is 15 milligrams. You easily can obtain
this amount of iron from a balanced diet that includes iron-rich foods. Table
A.5 on page 240 lists a number of vegan foods that are good sources of
iron. A few examples are soybeans, lentils, pumpkin seeds, spinach, and
dried peaches.

If you supplement your daily diet with a multivitamin/mineral, be careful that it does not contain more than 15 milligrams of iron, unless it has
been prescribed by your physician. Iron overload is called *hemochromato-
sis*. There are several ways that a person can become hemochromatic; too
much dietary and supplemental iron is one of them. Iron overload can be
fatal, as it can cause heart failure. Pituitary failure, abdominal pain, and
arthritis are also symptoms of iron overload.

ZINC

Zinc is another mineral that is fundamentally important for proper body functioning. It is a required part of more than seventy enzymes. Zinc also plays important roles in the immune functions of white blood cells, in amino acid metabolism, in lipid transport, and in the body's growth and development.

Factors That Affect Zinc Levels

The first cases of zinc deficiency were noted in the 1960s, in growing children and adolescent males living in Iran, Turkey, and Egypt. Their diets consisted of little meat and were high in whole grains (especially unleavened bread, in which the phytate had not been broken down) and beans. This eventually led to the conclusion that vegetarians are at risk for zinc deficiency, since their diets are usually rich in whole grains.

Zinc *is* found abundantly in meat products and it is believed that the body better absorbs zinc from meat than from plant substances. Since meat is noted as the main source of zinc in the Western diet, many vegetarians are warned that they are putting themselves at risk. But as this section will explain, a vegetarian diet is more than capable of providing a healthy amount of this mineral. Being aware of the factors that influence zinc absorption can help you make dietary decisions that will allow adequate levels. The main factors are phytate and calcium.

Phytate (especially from legumes) has been said to inhibit zinc absorption. Vegetarian diets are high in phytate, but if enough zinc is consumed, the vegetarian can maintain a healthy level. Researcher Freeland-Graves and colleagues published a study in 1980 that measured the zinc status of vegetarians. They found that the vegetarian women's poor dietary choices placed them at increased risk for poor zinc status. However, they also concluded that "vegetable protein foods can provide adequate amounts of zinc if consumed in large enough quantities." Therefore, more emphasis should be placed on encouraging vegetarian women to specifically eat foods that are rich sources of zinc in order to meet their nutrient needs.

It is encouraging to note that another study, performed by Anderson and colleagues, published in 1981, revealed that long-term vegetarians with high phytate consumption maintained healthy levels of zinc in their bodies. According to these researchers, the long-term vegetarians' bodies have adapted by increasing absorption of zinc. Furthermore, vegans who consume large amounts of whole grains and other zinc-rich plant foods, as well as modest amounts of calcium, are not at the increased risk of zinc deficiency at which other vegetarians who consume large amounts of calcium through milk and dairy foods are. Phytate seems to decrease zinc absorption primarily in the presence of calcium.

Suggested Intake and Sources of Zinc

For 11- to 51+-year-old females, the RDA for zinc is 12 milligrams. This is a minimum requirement. Again, the vegetarian female *can* obtain adequate zinc from food sources that are compatible with a vegetarian/vegan diet. For a list of zinc-rich vegan foods, see Table A.11 on page 244. Some examples are adzuki beans, sesame kernels, miso (a soyfood), and wheat germ. If you take a daily multivitamin/mineral, be sure it contains at least 50 percent of the RDA for zinc.

A diet that is low in zinc can cause numerous health problems. These include: diarrhea; hair loss; growth retardation; night blindness; poor appetite; changes in the sense of taste; and slow wound healing. Consult a physician if you are experiencing any of these signs.

VITAMIN B$_{12}$

Vitamin B$_{12}$ is necessary for the performance of three major bodily functions: the maintenance of the myelin sheaths that surround nerve fibers; the production of red blood cells by folate; and the activity and metabolism of bone cells. Vitamin B$_{12}$ is a difficult vitamin because it is found almost exclusively in animal flesh and animal products. So when it comes to arguing against a vegan diet, vitamin B$_{12}$ is the nutrient of target.

Vitamin B$_{12}$ Without Meat

Pro-meat-eaters insist that the vitamin B$_{12}$ issue is evidence that animal products are a necessary component of the human diet. What is the source of vitamin B$_{12}$ in animal products? Microorganisms in animals produce the vitamin B$_{12}$. But microorganisms are not only found in animals; they can contaminate any type of food, and they are also found in the soil. Therefore, oddly enough, contaminated food or water ends up being a source of vitamin B$_{12}$. Better sanitation measures have resulted in less contaminated food in the United States, and organizations are also working on cleaning the water. As a result, our vitamin B$_{12}$ supply is getting smaller.

Since vitamin B$_{12}$ is not naturally found in plant foods, how is it that there are hardly any cases of this deficiency in long-term vegans? That's a challenging question for researchers and health professionals. One reason is mentioned above; vegans get some vitamin B$_{12}$ from contaminated food and water. Another reason may be that vegans somehow efficiently conserve, absorb, and reuse previous stores of vitamin B_{12}. In addition, many products are now fortified with vitamin B_{12}. Finally, many vegans take vitamin B_{12} supplements, in which the vitamin is provided by yeast.

Suggested Intake and Sources of Vitamin B_{12}

Since a vitamin B_{12} deficiency can lead to serious problems, including irreversible nerve damage and paralysis, vegans should not gamble with their health. To ensure an adequate intake of this vitamin, take supplements or consume fortified vegan foods. For adult females, the RDA for vitamin B_{12} is 2.4 micrograms per day. The inclusion of any of the food products listed in Table A.8 on page 243, or other foods fortified with vitamin B_{12}, easily can meet the suggested daily intake. Examples of vegetarian sources of vitamin B_{12} include *EdenSoy Extra Soymilk* and Kellogg's *Total Whole Grain* cereal. If you do not purchase fortified foods, a multivitamin that includes vitamin B_{12} is strongly recommended.

VITAMIN D

Vitamin D has several main functions in the body. First, it maintains levels of calcium and phosphorus in the blood. Second, it is essential for the modeling and remodeling of bone. And finally, it promotes bone mineralization. Of all of the nutrients, vitamin D is the only one that can be supplied through exposure to the sun. The irradiation of the sun activates steroids in the skin that lead to the production of this nutrient. This makes vitamin D unique; it is not necessarily dependent upon dietary intake.

Vitamin D helps to increase the absorption of dietary calcium from the gastrointestinal tract. An inadequate intake of vitamin D or a depravation of sunlight will result in a withdrawal of calcium from the bones. Vitamin D deficiency causes *rickets,* which involves a bowing of the legs. It also results in *osteomalacia,* which is a softening of the bones.

Factors That Affect Vitamin D Levels

Certain individuals are at high risk of vitamin D deficiency due to inadequate sun exposure. Among these are people who live in cities with heavy smog, such as exists in areas of southern California. Environmental pollutants, including smog, block the sun's rays. Also, individuals who live in regions of the world that receive little sun exposure during certain months or seasons are at risk. The winter months in the northeastern areas of the

United States are characterized by little sunshine. An inadequate vitamin D intake is likely to occur during these months.

People who wear heavy clothing or do not expose their bodies to the sun have a good chance of being vitamin D deficient. Individuals who are home-bound often have this problem. It is also important to realize that in order to meet their vitamin D requirements, darker-skinned people need to stay out in the sun longer than fair-skinned people.

Suggested Intake and Sources of Vitamin D

The Adequate Intake (AI) for vitamin D is 5 micrograms per day. We have several options, since vitamin D can be supplied in three ways for vegans/vegetarians: through fortified foods; through supplementation; and through exposure to sunlight.

Nonvegan vegetarians can select milks and margarines that have been fortified with vitamin D, but the vegan has to turn to other sources. Substitute milk products, such as soymilk, soy drinks, and rice milk, are the most commonly fortified vegan foods. For example, 8 fluid ounces of a milk substitute—such as *West Brae, White Wave Silk Soymilk,* and *Rice Dream* products—provide a healthy dose of vitamin D. Another choice is fortified dry cereals. For a list of several vitamin D-fortified vegan foods, see Table A.10 on page 244. If these items don't please you, taking vitamin D supplements are an easy option.

The most significant source of vitamin D throughout the world is sunlight exposure. One excellent reason for obtaining your vitamin D from sunlight is that you do not have to worry about getting too much. The body has its own special mechanisms that protect against vitamin D intoxication. You can reach a healthy vitamin D level by spending approximately twenty to thirty minutes in the sun, three times a week.

When it comes to health, no one is exempt from carefully balancing nutrition. But it is not as difficult or intimidating as it first may seem—not even on a vegetarian or, moreover, a vegan diet. Consuming *at least* Dietary Reference Intake values for all nutrients is possible on a balanced vegetarian/vegan diet that includes some fortified foods (especially vitamin B_{12}-fortified foods) and adequate sunlight. (For more information on DRIs, see page 65.) Supplementation is also a part of maintaining a balanced diet. The next chapter will specifically discuss why supplementing with certain vitamins and minerals may help you to enhance your health.

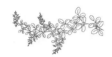 Chapter 6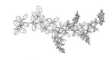

A Case for Supplementation

*Linda Tailor, a vegetarian of twenty-three years, was constantly hearing con-
flicting reports about whether or not supplements should be taken. She knew
it was not a good idea to take megadoses of vitamins and minerals, but Linda
also felt that some supplementation might be a good idea. After all, the soil
in which many of our crops are grown is now depleted of minerals, and some
foods are processed and refined to the point of severe nutrient loss.*

*Linda decided to seek the professional advice of a dietitian who spe-
cialized in vegetarian nutrition. The dietitian organized a program that
suited Linda's individual preferences. Linda now feels comfortable with the
daily consumption of superior vegan foods (SVFs)—foods that are especially high in nutrient content—and a multivitamin/mineral.*

The debate surrounding the use of nutritional supplements is one of the
hottest debates among health professionals today. Those against the
use of vitamin and mineral supplements state that a well-balanced diet is
capable of supplying all of the nutrients that the body needs to function
normally. When you think about it, we *should* be able to obtain complete
nutrition from our meals. After all, nature offers us food to eat, not a bunch
of tiny pills. But considering the transport, storage, packaging, and processing of many foods on the market today, as well as the contamination
and depletion of the environments in which they are grown, it is a good
idea to enhance diet through supplementation. We can do so with pill supplements and/or superior vegan foods (SVFs).

SUPPORT FOR SUPPLEMENTATION

Norman Potter, in the nutritional textbook *Food Science*, reports that food processing can destroy many essential vitamins and minerals, such as vitamin C, thiamin, riboflavin, niacin, and other water-soluble nutrients. M.T. Jordan, in his book *Reflections*, further explains that up to 70 percent of the nutrients found in whole foods are depleted by the time the foods are transported, stored, purchased, prepared, and cooked. This information offers good support for supplementation.

Storage and Preparation of Foods

Shari Lieberman and Nancy Bruning's *The Real Vitamin & Mineral Book* discusses the long process of nutrient depletion that our foods undergo. Fruits and vegetables begin to lose their nutrients the moment that they are picked off the plant. Then they are often stored, shipped, stored again, possibly processed, stored in our own kitchens, cut and sliced, and finally cooked. What's left by then? In *The Right Dose: How to Take Vitamins & Minerals Safely,* Patricia Hausman states that up to 100 percent of the vitamin C in a given food item can be eliminated due to ordinary processes of storing, cutting, and cooking. Also, the water-soluble nutrients, which include but are not exclusive to thiamin, vitamin B_6, niacin, and riboflavin, are likely to be completely absent by the time we consume what we think are "whole foods." Supplements can make up for this depletion.

Top Soil Depletion

Another strong argument for vitamin and mineral supplementation lies in the fact that the top soil in which crops are grown is steadily declining. Top soil is the richest soil, containing organisms and minerals that are important to the healthy development of crops. Overuse of the land has resulted in depletion of top soil, and what's worse, the soil is then often artificially fertilized to replenish some of the missing factors. The artificial fertilizers add more sodium and provide less nutrition to the plants. So our natural foods are not as healthy as they once were. Taking supplements can contribute to replacing what is now lacking in many fruits and vegetables even *before* they are picked.

Chemical Contamination

Moreover, author M.T. Jordan, mentioned above, explains that chemical contamination permeates our food and water supply. This contamination comes from a number of sources: pollution; herbicides; pesticides; radiation; preservatives; arsenic; and specific metals and metallic elements such as lead, mercury, aluminum, and cadmium, just to name a few. These harmful substances are carcinogens, which promote oxidation of our cells. *Oxidation* involves a reaction between oxygen and another substance, leading to chemical changes. As a result of cellular oxidation, free radicals are produced and are very capable of doing damage to the body. Free radicals are linked to such diseases as cancer and cardiovascular disease. See "Are We Captive to Free Radicals?" on page 169 for more information.

Fortunately, many vitamins and minerals are *antioxidants,* which can quench the free radicals and prevent them from doing harm. So it is helpful to supplement with such vitamins and minerals for preventative reasons. Supplements can supply amounts of antioxidants that would be hard to obtain from a reasonable diet.

In summary, most of us are exposed to extensive air, water, and land pollution, and therefore have increased needs for disease-fighting nutrients. Furthermore, many of our foods are lacking sufficient nutrients, as a result of soil depletion and food production/preparation techniques. Finally, don't overlook the fact that the stressful cultural environment in which many of us are forced to work and live puts even greater demands on the body. All of these factors boil down to the fact that vitamin and mineral supplements can help our bodies survive healthfully in harmful surroundings.

DECIPHERING THE CONFUSING ACRONYMS AND TERMS

In the past, nutrition professionals compared an individual's vitamin/mineral intakes with those suggested by the Recommended Dietary Allowances (RDAs) to determine whether or not that person was receiving adequate nutrition. The RDAs established the levels of intake necessary to avoid deficiency of certain nutrients. In 1998, the RDAs were replaced with a new standard called the Dietary Reference Intakes (DRIs).

The DRIs were designed for a broader purpose than the old standard. They were established not only to prevent nutrient deficiencies, but also to prevent the onset of certain chronic diseases. The DRIs are composed of four different categories: the Estimated Average Requirement (EAR), the Recommended Dietary Allowance (RDA), the Adequate Intake (AI), and the Tolerable Upper Intake (UI).

The Recommended Daily Intakes (RDIs), formerly called the U.S. RDAs, are based on the 1968 Recommended Dietary Allowances (RDAs) of the National Academy of Science. They are used in food labeling. Finally, the Daily Reference Value (DV) is also found on labels and apply to children over 4 years of age and adults. They are based on a daily intake of 2,000 calories. The DV includes the following nutrients: total fat; saturated fat; cholesterol; total carbohydrate; dietary fiber; sodium; potassium; and protein.

When a health-care practitioner refers to *optimal intakes,* he or she is discussing levels of nutrients believed to be the intakes that are most likely associated with disease prevention and optimal health maintenance. Optimal intake levels take into account that the vitamins and minerals that we consume in our foods are not 100-percent absorbed by our bodies. Therefore, higher doses might be beneficial and/or necessary.

Let us take, for example, zinc. In *Advanced Nutrition and Human Metabolism,* Sara Hunt and James Groff inform us that the absorption of zinc can vary from 14 to 41 percent, depending on the type of dietary substances consumed. Even if the RDI of 15 milligrams is consumed in a given day, depending on the type of foods eaten during meals, we might absorb only from 2 to 5 milligrams of zinc. A health professional might, therefore, suggest consuming an optimal intake of up to 25 milligrams.

Another case for optimal intakes is found in the example of folate (folic acid). Roberta Duyff, in *The American Dietetic Association's Complete Food and Nutrition Guide,* states, "Health authorities advise that any woman capable of becoming pregnant should consume 400 micrograms of folic acid daily from fortified foods, vitamin supplements, or a combination of the two. This *in addition to* [emphasis added] the folate

Women's Particular Needs

Women should be especially aware of their vitamin and mineral intakes for a number of reasons. First, heavy menstrual cycles can lead to deficiencies that merit supplementation, as can strenuous physical activity. Also, women of childbearing age need to take extra precautions to consume adequate amounts of nutrients, especially since many females do not know they are pregnant during the most vital development stages of the fetus. Pregnant and breast-feeding females must ensure an adequate intake of all nutrients during these life-giving stages. Finally, women who tend to have small appetites/intakes or who restrict their intakes for weight purposes are more likely to be consuming inadequate amounts of nutrients from their food choices.

found naturally in foods such as some fruits, vegetables, and legumes. This offers a safeguard against spinal cord defects in a developing fetus." If your health-care professional recommends an optimal intake for folate, you will be more likely to obtain the amount necessary for preventive measures.

Optimal intake levels are also designed to take into account factors such as environmental contamination and emotional stress. These factors can increase your needs for certain nutrients. Optimal intakes further establish the importance of taking supplements.

Table A.1 on page 234 gives the DRI/RDI and the optimal intake levels for vitamins and minerals. While the megadosing of nutrients is not recommended, taking a multivitamin/mineral supplement that contains close to 100 percent of the U.S. RDA in addition to a well-balanced vegan diet that aims to meet the RDA/RDI is strongly recommended.

NUTRIENTS IN A PILL OR ON THE PLATE?

When you hear the word *supplements,* the first thing that probably comes to mind is a cabinet jammed with bottles of colorful multivitamins and a varied collection of individual nutrients like vitamins B_{12} and C. However, supplementation does not refer only to nutrients in the form of pills; there are a variety of foods that vegans can use to reinforce their diets. The word supplement is defined by Webster's Dictionary as "referring to something added to supply a need or to reinforce." Reinforcement simply means to strengthen.

Pill Supplements

As a general rule of thumb, if you choose to use pill supplements *and* are eating a healthy vegetarian diet, I suggest that you select a pill supplement that offers supplementation closest to the amounts recommended by the DRIs (see page 65 for an explanation of DRIs). If you are consuming a healthy diet, you are probably already consuming at least 75 percent of the DRIs. Thus, a pill supplement that goes *way* beyond the DRIs is not necessary. This, of course, applies to individuals who have not been diagnosed with specific medical conditions that would merit greater intakes. A healthy diet will provide a good deal of individual nutrients; getting the majority of your nutrition through pills is neither necessary nor desirable.

Unfortunately, most vegan pill supplements contain an excess amount of the required dosages for adults. For example, I have yet to find a vegan multivitamin that contains only 2.4 micrograms—or 100 percent—of the DRI for vitamin B_{12}. The ones that I have come across contain anywhere from 48 to 250 micrograms! We are not really in danger of accumulating toxic levels of vitamin B_{12}; I use this only as an example. But keep in mind that in addition to the supplement, you will be accumulating nutrients from your food. So you don't want to overdose on some of the "more risky" nutrients, such as vitamin D, iron, vitamin A, and zinc. Children are more vulnerable to the dangers of over-supplementation, but all of us are at risk. Consider the information in Table 6.1.

Table 6.1. Toxicity Information on Selected Nutrients		
Vitamin/Mineral	**Toxic Dosage**	**Toxic Symptoms**
Vitamin A	More than 50,000 IU damage, and more.	Headache, blurred vision, nausea, vomiting, mouth dryness, bone abnormalities, liver
Vitamin D	More than 1,800 IU	Nausea, headache, diarrhea, fatigue, dizziness, loss of appetite, kidney stone formation.
Calcium	More than 3,000 mg	Inhibition of intestinal absorption of iron, zinc, and other essential minerals.
Iron	More than 75 mg	High toxic accumulations of iron can result in hemochromatosis. This is a dangerous condition that can lead to damage of the following organs, among others: liver, pancreas, and heart. (It's more common in children.) Nausea, vomiting, diarrhea, rapid heartbeat, weak pulse, dizziness, shock, confusion, death.
Zinc	2,000 mg or more	Gastrointestinal irritation, vomiting, dizziness, anemia, impaired immune response, impaired copper absorption.

If you are looking for a vegan multivitamin, I most highly recommend *MegaFood One Daily DailyFoods.* Other brands that I suggest include: *Natrol—My Favorite Multiple Take One; Living Source-Master; Nutrient System* by Rainbow Light; *Just One* by Rainbow Light; *Solgar Earth Source; Omnium-Solgar;* and *Solgar-Vegicaps Vegetarian Multiple.*

Now that the dangers of overdosing on pill supplements have been covered, it is necessary to state that, for most people, vitamin/mineral pill supplementation is a very healthy, beneficial part of the daily routine. Taking supplements that contain numerous antioxidants will help the body in its fight against free radicals. And balancing out your food nutrients with pill supplements can make all the difference when it comes to getting optimal intakes.

Superior Vegan Foods (SVFs)

The truth is that most of us find the convenience of pill supplements to be too handy to pass up. Many people are pressed for time and do not necessarily research and purchase food items that can serve as daily supplements. But if you are interested, there are several reasons why foods that are especially nutrient-dense, called superior vegan foods (SVFs), are an excellent alternative to—and possibly even more beneficial than—pill supplements:

- SVFs contain numerous vitamins and minerals that pill supplements do not contain, as well as other nutrients and compounds known to fight disease. For example, phytochemicals are health-enhancing plant chemicals.

- You are more likely to take toxic doses of single nutrients through pill supplements than you are through SVFs.

- Food supplements are usually less expensive than pill supplements.

- Some pill supplements do not properly dissolve in the digestive tract. Therefore, the benefits are not reaped. Unless you have a gastrointestinal condition, SVFs will be digested well and you will receive all of the nutritional advantages.

- Pill supplements can be difficult to swallow. And quite simply, foods taste better!

What exactly is an SVF? For the *vegan female,* I define an SVF as a nutrient-dense food to which any of the following apply (the references to

Table 6.2. Superior Vegan Foods

Food	Main Nutrient Contents
Adzuki beans, boiled (1 cup)	4.60 mg iron; 120 mg magnesium; 385 mg phosphorus; 0.27 mg thiamin; 4.06 mg zinc.
Blackstrap molasses (2 tbsp)	344 mg calcium; 7 mg iron; 86 mg magnesium.
Brewer's yeast (1 oz)	4.90 mg iron; 10.70 mg niacin; 497 mg phosphorus; 1.21 mg riboflavin; 4.43 mg thiamin.
Collard greens, frozen (1 cup)	358 mg calcium; 130 mcg folate; 638 RE (retinol equivalents) vitamin A; 46 mg vitamin C.
Figs (10 dried)	269 mg calcium; 4.18 mg iron; 111 mg magnesium; 0.42 milligrams vitamin B_6.
Garbonzo beans/chickpeas, boiled (1 cup)	282 mcg folate ; 4.74 mg iron; 78.00 mg magnesium; 275 mg phosphorus.
Great Northern beans, canned (1 cup)	213 mcg folate; 4.11 mg iron; 134 mg magnesium; 355 mg phosphorus; 0.38 mg thiamin.
Lentils, boiled (1 cup)	358 mcg folate; 6.59 mg iron; 356 mg phosphorus; 0.34 mg thiamin.
Natto ($\frac{1}{2}$ cup)	7.57 mg iron; 101 mg magnesium; 153 mg phosphorus.
Navy beans, boiled (1 cup)	255 mcg folate; 4.51 mg iron; 107 mg magnesium; 285 mg phosphorus; 0.37 mg thiamin.
Red kidney beans, boiled (1 cup)	229 mcg folate; 5.20 mg iron; 80 mg magnesium; 252 mg phosphorus; 0.28 mg thiamin.
Red Star Nutritional Yeast ($1\frac{1}{2}$ to 2 tsp)	2 mcg vitamin B_{12}.
Soy nuts ($\frac{1}{2}$ cup)	232 mg calcium; 176 mg folate; 3.40 mg iron; 196 mg magnesium; 558 mg phosphorus; 0.65 mg riboflavin; 0.37 mg thiamin; 4.10 mg zinc.

Food	Main Nutrient Contents
Soybeans, boiled (1 cup)	8.84 mg iron; 421 mg phosphorus; 0.49 mg riboflavin; 0.27 mg thiamin; .4 mg vitamin B_6.
Tortula yeast (1 ounce)	5.50 mg iron; 12.60 mg niacin; 486 mg phosphorus; 1.43 mg riboflavin; 3.97 mg thiamin.
Whole fruit/vegetable juices (1 cup)	Several nutrients, depending on types of fruits/vegetables used.

groups 1, 2, and 3 apply to the boxed information given below): a vegan food that contains at least two nutrients from the group 1 and group 2 nutrients, and moreover, at least 25 percent of the daily requirement of these nutrients for 21- to 50-year-old females; a vegan food that contains one of the nutrients from group 3; a fortified vegan food that contains all of the group 1 and group 3 nutrients, as well as many nutrients from group 2.

Group 1 nutrients: iron; calcium; folic acid (folate); zinc.

Group 2 nutrients: other vitamins/minerals: vitamin A; vitamin E; vitamin K; vitamin C; thiamin; riboflavin; niacin; vitamin B_6; phosphorus; magnesium; iodine; selenium.

Group 3 nutrients: vitamin B_{12}; vitamin D.

Table 6.2 provides a list of superior vegan foods. The amounts of the main nutrients that each food contains are also identified.

In addition, the following are examples of vegan *fortified* foods that serve as food supplements: *General Mill's Total* cereal; *Kellogg's Product 19* cereal; *Green Giant Breakfast Patties; Green Giant Harvest Burgers; EdenSoy Extra Soymilk;* and *Worthington's Tuno.*

WHAT'S RIGHT FOR YOU?

What is the optimal amount of vitamins or minerals that *you* should ingest? Each and every human being on this earth is designed differently. These differences make it difficult to make only one set of recommendations. All of us cannot fit under the same umbrella. If we try, those of us who are taller will stay dry, while those of us who are shorter will get wet. You must take a look at your very specific lifestyle, habits, environment, and genetic make-up in order to determine what is right for you.

Take, for example, a female marathon runner; this individual will need extra iron because marathon runners tend to develop iron deficiency anemia due to their strenuous routines. Or consider someone who has a habit of smoking; a smoker actually needs to increase vitamin C intake to almost double the amount required for a non-smoker. Individuals who have certain disease processes might need larger amounts of certain nutrients. If you have a condition that increases your need for specific vitamins and minerals, consult a health professional for medical advice. Actually, it is a good idea for every individual to work with a nutritionist on finding what levels of vitamins and minerals are optimal for her specific body.

The purpose of this chapter is not to sell you on supplements. I simply would like you to think about the environment in which you live and to answer this question for yourself: "Is it possible for me to live an optimally healthy life without some type of supplementation?" Remember, supplementation does not necessarily involve taking several "horse bullets" every day. SVFs can adequately enhance your diet and bring you to a healthier state, if you so choose. But it is a good idea to take some form of a daily supplement, as it will help to ensure that you are receiving a complete regimen of the nutrients that may be lacking in today's food supply.

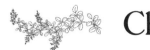 # Chapter 7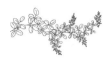

The Vegetarian Adolescent

Barbara Thompson and her parents decided to become vegans when Barbara was 14 years old. Quite a number of people criticized Barbara for choosing veganism right at the time of her growth spurt. Rumors circulated that her growth would be stunted, that she would be anemic, and that she would surely have bone problems later in life. However, Barbara's family did the necessary research on how to follow veganism. They consumed well-balanced meals and took proper supplementation. When Barbara hit 19 years of age, she was 5'7" tall, which is two inches over the median for the reference female in the United States. She weighed 135 pounds, which placed her at an appropriate weight for her height and build. Barbara was active, happy, and on the road to a lifetime of optimal health.

Today, many teens are deciding to become vegetarians on their own, without the influence and sometimes without the support of parents. They are finding that a vegetarian diet helps them to control their weight, increases their vigor and energy, and keeps them looking and feeling healthy. In addition, as increased numbers of teens become aware of the cruel treatment of food animals, many choose to express their feelings and make positive changes by following a vegetarian diet. This commitment to a meatless diet has raised concern within the traditional American family that is used to sitting down to a hearty meat-based dinner.

It might not be difficult for an adolescent to decide to become a vegetarian. But does she know *how* to follow a vegetarian diet properly? Does she know what foods she must consume to ensure an adequate intake of nutrients during her growth and development? This chapter will address these concerns. But first, let's discuss the ways that vegetarianism can add to the immediate and long-term health of adolescent girls.

ADVANTAGES OF VEGETARIAN ADOLESCENTS

Adolescents who are raised vegetarian or who choose to become vegetarian can experience extra health advantages. They have a tendency for healthier body weight and also increase their chances of preventing the onset of chronic disease. I am sure no one will argue with me when I say that it is more beneficial and cost-effective to keep your car in good shape than it is to fix it after it breaks down. We should apply the same system of thought to our bodies. A healthy dietary regimen during adolescence could make all the difference in later life.

Better Weight Control

Obesity among adolescents has become an increasing problem in our society. Statistics estimate that 10 to 25 percent of American teenagers are obese. Furthermore, 80 percent of overweight teens will become overweight adults. These facts shouldn't surprise us, considering the amount of high-fat and high-calorie foods readily available to the American population. But vegetarian youths are less likely to be obese. That means that they are reducing their risk of certain chronic diseases, such as cardiovascular disease and diabetes.

The negative health effects of obesity are profound. A follow-up to a long-term Harvard Growth Study was published by the *New England Journal of Medicine* in 1992. It looked at the relationship between obesity and disease/death rate in 508 participants. The subjects were first recorded as lean or overweight adolescents when they were aged 13 to 18 years. Their health was then tracked into their senior years. The researchers found that the disease rate from coronary heart disease and atherosclerosis was increased among men and women who had been overweight in adolescence. Furthermore, the incidence of arthritis was increased among women who had been overweight teenagers. The researchers concluded that being overweight in the teen years can lead to many adverse health effects in adulthood.

Habits formed in childhood and adolescence that are not corrected can lead to regrets in adulthood. When an obese or overweight adolescent loses excess weight, he or she dramatically improves in health status. Parents need to encourage and teach their children how to eat to live, instead of how to live to eat. One way to do this is to promote a vegetarian diet.

A vegetarian diet planned in the proper way is both low in fat and high in complex carbohydrates, including fiber. These are two dietary aspects that encourage healthy weight, thus decreasing the risk of coronary heart disease, atherosclerosis, arthritis, and diabetes. Diabetes, in particular, is a very real problem for many adolescents. In a 1999 article from *Clinical Insights in Diabetes #2,* the National Diabetes Education Initiative reported that type 2 diabetes has reached epidemic proportions in adolescents. A third of the new cases of diabetes is occurring in individuals 10 to 20 years of age. This epidemic is associated with obesity. For more information on obesity, see Chapter 14.

Recently there have been reports that vegetarianism plays a role in eating disorders, since some teens turn to a vegetarian diet to help control their weight. However, eating disorders are psychological diseases; food is simply the medium through which the victims feel that they express control. Vegetarianism is not the culprit. Any diet (meat-based or vegetarian) can be used in a harmful manner.

Later Onset of Puberty

The first menstrual period is called menarche. It is true that the age of menarche has been found to occur later in vegetarian girls. In a study published in 1992, Sabate and colleagues reported that lacto-ovovegetarian girls experienced menarche about six months later than meat-eating girls in the same geographical area.

As explained in Neal Barnard's *Food for Life,* Dr. T. Colin Campbell, a biochemist at Cornell University, directed a massive China Health Study and found that the age of puberty in Chinese girls averaged at 17 years. Quite differently, the average American girl begins puberty as she nears or turns 11 years of age. Asian cuisines are recognized for their high-soy and low-meat content. It is not unreasonable to suspect that the emphasis on plant foods influences age of menarche.

In the *American Journal of Clinical Nutrition,* Kinsella reported that with the Westernization of the Japanese diet, there was a drop in the onset of puberty from slightly over 15 years to 12.5 years of age. The Westernization of the Japanese diet involves changing from a diet rich in soy and other plant foods to a diet that is high in fat and low in fiber. Meat, dairy products, and eggs are staples of typical Western cuisine. From this study and the one mentioned above, we can surmise that a vegetarian diet may delay certain aspects of maturation in some girls. However, it is important to realize that these delays are likely to have long-term advantages, possibly carrying positive health benefits into adulthood. A later age of menarche has consistently been associated with decreased risk for several cancers, particularly breast cancer.

VEGETARIANISM AND ADOLESCENT GROWTH

If you are worried about whether or not a vegetarian, and moreover a vegan diet can support the growth spurts of adolescence, you are not alone. This is a common concern. In fact, misinformation has circulated that vegetarianism stunts growth. I can truthfully tell you that a balanced, meatless diet can certainly provide optimal nutrition and support adolescent growth. Remind yourself that vegetarianism has been practiced by many people throughout history. Countless children have been successfully raised on vegetarian diets. In addition, scientific studies were conducted to investigate this very worry.

A study involving 1,765 children was conducted by Sabate, Linsted, Harris, and Sanchez and published in 1991. Of the participants, 895 were meat-eaters and 870 were vegetarians; 886 were female and 879 were male. The researchers found that all of the vegetarian children scored higher than the fiftieth percentile on the National Center for Health Statistics, and that they were actually taller than their meat-eating contemporaries. These results did not change when parental height and socioeconomic factors were taken into consideration for a subsample of 518 children. The researchers concluded that, "vegetarian children and adolescents on a balanced diet grow at least as tall as children who consume meat."

A 1992 study, done by Sabate, Llorca, and Sanchez, looked solely at the heights of 11- to 12-year-old vegetarian and nonvegetarian children. The research showed that the heights of the vegetarian girls were about 3 centimeters less than their meat-eating counterparts. However, the vegetarian girls continued to grow and reached final heights similar to those of the meat-eaters. No significant differences between the two groups were found. The initial lower height of the vegetarian girls may be indicative of a later onset of puberty or a delayed onset of pubertal growth.

THE DEMAND FOR NUTRIENTS DURING FEMALE ADOLESCENCE

Adolescence is a very special time for every female. The body goes through many physical changes as a girl blossoms into a mature woman. The adolescent growth spurt for females begins between the ages of 10.5 and 11 years, and peaks at the age of 12.

The adolescent first experiences an increase in height. Females grow approximately six inches during this time. The skeletal system undergoes

More Support for a Meatless Youth

If you are still having doubts, perhaps recent professional support will do the trick. More and more people within the health fields are stating that a carefully planned and followed vegetarian diet can provide the nutritional needs of both children and adolescents. The *American Journal of Clinical Nutrition* fully supports a vegetarian diet for adolescents: "There is no doubt that a properly selected vegetarian diet can meet all the requirements of growing children. . . ." Furthermore, the *American Dietetic Association* revealed its support of vegetarianism for young people when it stated, "Infants, children, and adolescents who consume well planned vegetarian diets can generally meet all of their nutritional requirements for growth." This organization also endorses veganism.

Veganism is as capable as any other vegetarian and meat-based diet. Dr. Reed Mangels, a registered dietitian with a doctorate degree in nutrition and also the former President of the American Dietetic Association's Vegetarian Practice Group, wrote an excellent article entitled "Feeding Vegan Kids." It is published in Mangels' and Wasserman's *Simply Vegan*. In it, Mangels confirms that *vegan* children can attain adequate health and growth and maintain very high levels of activity. Furthermore, Mangels reminds us that while it may take time and work to feed a vegan child, isn't it true that providing a balanced diet for *any* child means committing your time and thoughts?

tremendous change as the bones lengthen and the epiphyses—the ends of the long bones—finally close. Thirty-five pounds is the average amount of weight that most females gain during this growth spurt. Hormones that control the secondary sexual characteristics drastically increase and, as a result, the ovaries grow, the breasts enlarge, pubic hair appears, and menstruation begins.

Normal development and good nutrition go hand in hand. Adequate protein and calories are critical in order for any type of growth to occur. Keep in mind the fact that no matter how much protein is eaten, growth cannot occur normally if the intake of energy-providing (calorie-supplying) nutrients—carbohydrates and fats—is too low. In addition, proper mineral intake is essential to health. The adolescent will need more calcium to support her bone growth. The start of her menstrual flow will increase her need for iron. With all of this in mind, let us discuss the adolescent's changing nutrient needs and how they can be met on a vegetarian/vegan diet.

Carbohydrates, Fats, and Protein

Carbohydrates and fats are the two main contributors of calories in the diet. *Both* are necessary. Carbohydrates are generally defined as sugars, starches, and fiber. They provide glucose, which is the body's main source of energy. Whole grains and fruits are the major sources of carbohydrates. Adolescents should try to follow the recommended number of servings suggested in Table 4.2 on page 47.

Fat is also a critical nutrient that performs essential functions in the body, including: protection of internal organs from damage; insulation of the body; maintenance of normal body temperature; aid in transporting fat-soluble nutrients; and help in maintaining the health and structure of the body's cells. Some adolescents choose a vegetarian diet because they are trying to abstain from fat, and a meatless diet is naturally lower in fat. What teens must understand is that fat is a *necessary* part of a healthy diet—the body cannot function properly without it. The best sources of dietary fat include nuts and seeds, soft margarines, and oils like canola and olive oils, instead of stick margarines and butter.

Protein's fundamental role in health and development is discussed in Chapters 4 and 5. Protein intake is basic to proper growth and muscular development. It is also essential to the maintenance of healthy digestion, body fluid balance, immunity, and hormone activity.

Table 7.1 gives the Recommended Dietary Allowances for protein and calories for females in two different age groups. Remember that each individual is different, and that a child's needs may differ from the general recommendations. The best indicator that a teen is receiving adequate nutrition is her continued growth, maintenance of a healthy body weight, and good energy levels. If the adolescent is not adequately growing, you should seek the advice of a health professional such as a dietitian.

The protein and calorie levels listed on page 79 are general estimates; the recommended calorie levels may promote obesity in some adolescents. While an adequate caloric intake is essential, obesity is undesirable. If an adolescent is gaining an unhealthy amount of weight or is already overweight, a lower calorie intake is recommended.

Minerals

Two minerals of special concern for the female adolescent are calcium and iron. Both of these minerals are traditionally areas of concern for vegetari-

Weight in Pounds	RDAs for 11- to 14-Year-Olds		RDAs for 15- to 18-Year-Olds	
	Protein (g)	Calories	Protein (g)	Calories
80	36	1,692	29	1,440
85	39	1,833	31	1,560
90	41	1,927	33	1,640
95	43	2,021	34	1,720
100	45	2,115	36	1,818
105	48	2,256	38	1,920
110	50	2,350	40	2,000
115	52	2,444	42	2,080
120	55	2,585	44	2,200
125	57	2,679	46	2,280
130	59	2,773	47	2,360
135	61	2,867	49	2,440
140	64	3,008	51	2,560

Table 7.1. Protein and Calorie Requirements for Female Adolescents

ans, as well. But as explained in Chapter 5, the vegetarian diet (including the vegan diet) is completely capable of providing optimal mineral intakes.

Calcium

Calcium is especially important for proper bone development. It is during adolescence that the rate of bone formation predominates over the rate of resorption. In other words, bone is being formed at an accelerated rate. During childhood growing years, about 140 to 165 milligrams of calcium per day are used. During the pubertal growth period, possibly up to 400 to 500 milligrams of calcium per day are used. Therefore, is it vital that adolescents meet their requirements for this mineral.

The recommended calcium intake for females aged 9 to 19 years is 1,300 milligrams per day. As mentioned in Chapter 5, vegetarians have lower calcium needs than meat-eaters, due to their lower protein intake. However, since the calcium requirement for vegetarians has not specifically been established, it would be a good idea to shoot for the current recommendations.

A good knowledge of calcium-rich vegan foods will help teens meet their required needs. While adolescents may not want to get their calcium from collard greens or blackstrap molasses, they might settle for foods such as *White Wave Dairyless Yogurt* or other soy yogurts, fortified soy/oat/rice beverages, calcium-fortified orange juice, raisins, soynuts, and *Soymage* cheese. For a list of calcium-rich vegan foods, see Table A.2 on page 236.

Iron

Menarche, or the commencement of the menstrual flow, directly affects iron status. This is because iron is stored in a molecule called *hemoglobin,* which is a component of blood. When a girl starts her period, the loss of blood results in a reduced iron level. In addition to the changes that occur with the menstrual cycle, adolescents require more iron as their physical growth increases.

The Recommended Dietary Allowance (RDA) for iron for 11- to 18-year-old females is 15 milligrams per day. *Keep in mind that this suggestion is a minimum intake.* Female adolescents are more likely than males to suffer from iron deficiency anemia. The Second National Health and Nutrition Examination Survey (NHANES II) of the United States population found that 5 percent of females aged 15 to 19 years had impaired iron status.

If all meat-eating female adolescents are not consuming adequate iron to meet their needs (even though they are supposedly eating the best source of iron), what about vegetarian teenage girls? Research by Nelson and associates, published in 1994, included 114 schoolgirls aged 11 to 14 years. The researchers found that 20 percent of the girls had low hemoglobin. A low hemoglobin level can be an indicator of poor iron stores. They then tracked the incidence of low hemoglobin among the vegetarians in the group, and found it was 20 percent. The conclusion was there was no difference in the prevalence of low hemoglobin between nonvegetarians, as a group, and vegetarians, as a group.

The vegetarian adolescent should be sure to eat a variety of foods that are rich in iron, such as dark green, leafy vegetables. Iron-rich foods should be eaten with foods or juices that contain vitamin C, since that vitamin increases the absorption of iron. Please refer to page 240 for a list of vegan iron-rich foods, and page 243 for a list of vitamin C-rich foods.

The adolescent athlete has several additional needs. For information, see Chapter 8, pages 91 to 92. Also, keep in mind that the pregnant or lactating adolescent female has greater nutritional requirements. For information, see Chapter 9, pages 106 to 107.

DAILY MEAL PATTERN GUIDELINES FOR VEGAN ADOLESCENTS

The vegan adolescent should generally follow the food pattern guidelines offered in Table 4.2 on page 47. In order to meet her calcium requirements, the adolescent vegan should include one to two servings of foods that contain more than 200 milligrams of calcium per serving. For example, 1 to 2 cups of calcium-fortified orange juice can serve as one of her daily fruit servings, or 1 to 2 cups of calcium-fortified soymilk/soy drink (containing at least 20 percent of the daily value for calcium) as one of her tofu/soy product servings. These should be taken in addition to other calcium-rich foods. Finally, the vegan adolescent should be sure to consume one to two servings of iron-rich legumes, vegetables, and other foods.

Table 7.2 on page 82 offers three sample daily menus; it lists practical meal plans at three different caloric levels. All three vegan plans provide more than 100 percent of the required protein for the specific calorie bracket and more than 100 percent of the general nutritional needs of an adolescent. The menus are constructed for 11- to 18-year-olds.

There are a few more things to consider in addition to the three meals of the day. For adequate vitamin-D intake, physical activity in the sunlight is strongly suggested. And, as most adolescents love to snack in-between meals, some nutritious noshes include: apple chips; dried fruit; crackers with peanut butter; crackers with tofu/*Tuno* dip; fresh fruit; nuts/seeds; popcorn with brewer's yeast; rice cakes; and vegetables with tofu/*Tuno* dip.

PARENTS' GUIDELINES FOR FOSTERING NUTRITION AWARENESS

Truly, adults have a responsibility to empower adolescents with nutritional knowledge. It is important to keep in mind that, when it comes to nutrition, what you put into your child's head is as important as what you put on her plate. Here are a few tips on how to get your teenager to become a disciplined and healthy eater.

* Outline the numerous diet-related diseases from which people suffer, and the foods that help cause these diseases. (See Part Three of this book for detailed information on diet and chronic diseases.)

Table 7.2. Sample Menus

Breakfast	Lunch	Dinner

1,800 Calorie Meal Plan

Breakfast	Lunch	Dinner
½ cup oatmeal	1 tofu-spinach patty sandwich	½ cup Spanish rice
1 whole wheat bagel	½ cup potato salad	½ cup Great Northern beans
1 tbsp almond butter	1 cup carrot sticks	½ cup collard greens
1 banana	6 oz calcium-fortified orange juice	1 whole wheat dinner roll
1 cup fortified soymilk		6 oz apple juice

2,200 Calorie Meal Plan

Breakfast	Lunch	Dinner
¾ cup granola sprinkled with 1 oz sunflower seeds	1 large bean burrito	1½ cups vegan-style scalloped potatoes
1 cup fortified soymilk	10 dried apple slices	1 cup turnip greens
3 vegan sausages	4 oz tofu pudding	1 slice garlic bread
1 banana muffin	1 cup calcium-fortified orange juice	1 cup garden salad
1 cup fruit salad		½ cup apricot nectar

2,500 Calorie Meal Plan

Breakfast	Lunch	Dinner
1 cup *Total* flakes	1 veggie-burger on whole wheat bun	1 cup macaroni and veggie-burger casserole
1 cup fortified soymilk	6 oz soy yogurt	1 cup broccoli/carrots steamed
4 oz scrambled tofu	1 oz mixed nuts	1 cup tossed spinach salad with 1 cup chickpeas
1 slice whole wheat toast	2 plums	1 tbsp homemade Italian salad dressing
1 tsp margarine	1 cup calcium-fortified orange juice	1 whole wheat dinner roll
1 pear or 10 dried figs		1 cup peach nectar

• Visit a hospital or a nursing home with your teen, and have a health-care professional explain the physical and mental consequences of diet-related diseases.

• Visit or speak with different health associations—for example, the American Heart Association, the Diabetes Association, the American Cancer Institute—with your teen and obtain literature from these associations that emphasizes a healthy, balanced diet.

• Order a Vegetarian Food Pyramid (see below the illusration on page 38) and post it in a visible place in the kitchen.

• Help your adolescent to draw up menus that meet her nutritional needs. Use the food pattern guide on page 47 and the sample menus on page 82 for help. Make her favorite healthy foods a significant part of her meal plan.

• Encourage your teen to try new vegan foods and to keep an open mind about unfamiliar foods.

• Teach your adolescent to cook; help her to become an active participant in the kitchen. Several excellent cookbooks are listed in Appendix B.

• Advise your child to join organizations like the Vegan Society for Teens. Such groups will provide strong support for her and will help her in making good choices. (See Appendix C for information on vegetarian organizations and resources.)

• Suggest that both of you read books and other literature that will help the family make the necessary adjustments that a vegetarian diet requires. Some recommended books are: *Vegetarian Children: A Supportive Guide for Parents* by Sharon Yntema; *A Teen's Guide to Going Vegetarian* by Judy Krizmanic; *Simply Vegan* by Debra Wasserman and Reed Mangels; and *Vegetables Rock!: A Complete Guide for Teenage Vegetarians* by Stephanie Pierson.

These activities will not only get your teen thinking about nutrition, but will also increase the quality time that you spend together. Change is most effective when people help each other to learn. You, too, will gain much knowledge about health and may end up making a few life-changing choices of your own.

Those adolescents who choose a vegetarian diet should feel confident that with some careful planning, they can meet their nutritional needs. They will find that vegetarianism is an excellent way to maintain and improve health, both in the present and in the future. Vegetarianism contributes to healthy weight control and the prevention of numerous chronic diseases. It encourages the female adolescent to feel good, in body and spirit.

It is important to realize that the health benefits of a vegetarian diet will be reaped only if the adolescent follows the vegetarian diet appropriately. If she simply avoids meat and does not substitute any other nutrient-dense foods, the health advantages of vegetarianism are lost. It will take some work to carve out a vegetarian plan that suits individual needs and life-stage requirements, but any healthy diet will demand such time and research. The benefits of vegetarianism, especially at a stage when the body is setting patterns for life, make the efforts worthwhile.

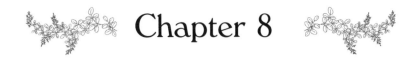

Chapter 8

The Physically Active Vegetarian

Surya Bonaly, born December 15, 1973, was already a world-recognized ice skater at the age of 15. In 1989, at the European Championship competition in Birmingham, England, she finished fourth in the free-skate. Later that year, Bonaly finished tenth in her World Championship debut. By 25 years of age, Surya had been a nine-time French National Champion 1988–1996), a five-time European Champion (1991–1995), a three-time World Silver Medalist (1993–1995), and a World Junior Champion (1991).

Bonaly was said to "rule her sport" in Europe. She is the only woman to perform a back flip on ice skates and land on just one foot. She is also a vegan. Surya's adoptive parents raised her on a strict vegetarian (macrobiotic) diet; she consumes no milk or other animal products. And from her performance and her appearance, it is obvious that Bonaly is in top physical condition.

Contrary to popular belief, a vegetarian diet *can* support the strenuous physical demands placed on the bodies of professional athletes, as well as the needs of females who regularly exercise for health and fitness. As a matter of fact, exercise and a vegetarian diet make a perfect match. The benefits promote physical, mental, and spiritual health. Both exercise and a vegetarian diet are associated with lowering the risk of many of the chronic diseases that are afflicting countless Americans today—obesity, diabetes, heart disease, and hypertension. This chapter will discuss exercise and how the vegetarian diet can support the active body.

THE BENEFITS OF EXERCISE

Exercise has become a very popular word in the American culture. We are bombarded with pressure to get more of it. And, to the delight of many health professionals, the number of exercising Americans has been increasing. Today, there are more than 22 million exercising women in the United States alone.

Physical activity has many beneficial effects on participants of all ages. For example, it:

- strengthens the cardiovascular system

- improves circulation

- increases physical strength

- strengthens the bones (aerobic exercise, such as walking and jogging)

- promotes weight loss

- improves diabetic control

- helps reduce high blood pressure

- reduces risk of atherosclerosis

- improves self-esteem

- relieves stress

With all of these benefits come increased demands on the body for more nutrients and calories (if weight loss is not desired). A properly planned and followed vegetarian diet can easily meet the nutritional needs of physically active women. Considering that we have so many examples of professional athletes who are vegetarians, there is no reason to question the adequacy of a meatless diet for exercising females.

Martina Navratilova, who was one of the world's top tennis players, is also a vegetarian athlete. Navratilova believes that her whole-foods diet, which consists of raw fruits and vegetables, rice, pasta, and a few grains, enabled her to extend her professional tennis career. Martina and Surya Bonaly (discussed at the beginning of this chapter) are only two of many examples. You will probably be amazed to find out that the following athletes are also vegetarians: Romy Karz, vegan ballerina; Sally Hibberd, British women's mountain bike champion; Debbie Lawrence, world record holder for the women's 5K race walk event; Kathy Johnson, Olympic silver medallist in gymnastics; Sharon Hounsell, Miss Wales Bodybuilding champion; Billie Jean King, tennis champion; Diana McCabe, distance runner; Lucy Stephens, vegan triathlete; and Spice Williams, vegan body-builder, actress, and stunt woman. Now isn't that an impressive list of vegetarians?

GUIDELINES FOR EXERCISE

It seems that exercise is one of those few situations in which more is better. Studies on female runners have shown that those who increase their mileage from ten miles a week to forty miles a week can reduce their risk of coronary heart disease by 29 percent. Yet we don't have to run forty miles—or even ten miles—a week to reap the benefits of exercise. According to Centers for Disease Control and Prevention (CDCP) and the American College of Sports Medicine (ACSM), "Every U.S. adult should accumulate 30 minutes or more of moderate-intensity physical activity on most, preferably all, days of the week." Each person can achieve this while doing the activity (or activities) that she likes most, such as swimming, bicycling, or taking a fun aerobics class.

The Nutrition Edition of the American Dairy Association & Dairy Council Mid East used an Activity Pyramid developed by Park Nicollet Medical Foundation to develop a healthy activity schedule for the week. They suggest that every day of the week, you should carry out basic physical activities whenever possible: walk the dog; take the stairs instead of the elevator; park your car farther away than you used to; work in the garden or on your lawn. Three to five times per week, take at least thirty minutes to perform a recreational activity that results in calorie burning, such as tennis, basketball, or dancing. Also three to five times per week, set aside at least twenty minutes for motivated aerobic activity, such as a fast walk, a swim, bicycling, or rollerblading. Activities that increase flexibility and strength, such as push-ups and weightlifting, should be performed two to three times a week. So should healthy leisure activities, like softball and bowling; during these games, you are not constantly exercising, but you do have periods of movement and stretching. Do not allow sedentary activities that have you sitting for more than thirty minutes—for example, watching TV, playing computer games—to take up much of your time.

Following the above-described plan will yield the benefits of regular exercise described previously in this chapter. If you are just starting out or are planning to change your regular exercise habits, remember that increases in exercise routines should be done gradually. Those with medical conditions (for example, heart disease) should consult their physicians before starting an exercise program.

FUELING EXERCISE

The three major fuel sources of the energy we use to move, exercise, and simply function are carbohydrates, fats, and proteins. The body relies mainly on carbohydrates and fats for its energy, with proteins making a smaller contribution at all times. These sources are converted to a molecule called *adenosine triphosphate,* more commonly referred to as *ATP.*

During the first thirty seconds of exercise, the muscles are able to obtain immediate fuel from small body stores of energy. After these stores are depleted, the body must obtain energy from other reservoirs. It is able to produce energy for another three minutes by converting carbohydrates to lactic acid. So, during the first few minutes of exercise, readily available stored resources are utilized. Anaerobic exercise—for example, sprinting, lifting weights—uses such stored energy and does not employ oxygen. It develops strength and increases bulk in the muscles.

Aerobic exercise, on the other hand, requires the use of oxygen. When we exercise aerobically, the body breaks into its stores of carbohydrates, fats, and proteins to meet its energy demands. Aerobic exercise takes place after about three minutes, when the initial energy stores are used up. This type of exercise strengthens our cardiovascular system and promotes weight loss. Examples of aerobic exercise are swimming, fast walking, jogging, basketball, and cross-country skiing.

Carbohydrates

Carbohydrates are the body's main energy source during anaerobic exercise. *Glycogen* is the storage form of carbohydrates and is stored in the muscles and the liver. The body is dependent upon glycogen; it is necessary for any type of physical activity to occur, whether anaerobic or aerobic. And the more glycogen stores available, the longer a person can exercise. Fatigue is the consequence of insufficient glycogen stores and is more likely to occur earlier if the muscle glycogen stores are small.

Diet directly affects glycogen stores. The more carbohydrates a physically active female eats, the larger the glycogen stores that she has available. Furthermore, intensity of exercise affects the use of these glycogen stores. High-intensity activities, such as sprinting, use up the glycogen stores more quickly than less intense activities, like jogging. A depletion of glycogen usually occurs within 90 to 120 minutes of vigorous or aerobic exercise.

For the physically active individual, it is recommended that carbohydrates contribute 60 to 65 percent of total energy intake. Whole grains such as whole wheat bread or bagels, cereals like oatmeal and *Whole Grain Total,* pastas, and starchy vegetables like potatoes are excellent sources of carbohydrates.

Fats

The body's supply of glycogen as an energy source seems small when compared with the virtually unlimited availability of body fat. The longer an individual aerobically exercises at a moderate intensity, the more fat will be used as fuel. Exercising for more than twenty minutes allows more fat and less glycogen to be used. In other words, if you want to lose body fat, perform aerobic exercise (even simply walking) at a moderate intensity for more than twenty minutes.

Fat should contribute no more than 30 percent of total energy intake. A low-fat diet is recommended to prevent and reduce the risk of heart disease. Furthermore, according to Rolfes and Debruyne's *Life Span Nutrition: Conception Through Life,* athletes on high-carbohydrate diets perform three times longer than those on high-fat diets. For athletes who have enormous calorie needs, after calculating the carbohydrate and protein requirements, fats can be used to provide additional calories. Nuts are an excellent source of additional calories, while also protecting against heart disease—their fats are mostly "good" fats. In addition, they provide protein and other nutrients.

Protein

Protein is also used as fuel during exercise, but to a much lesser extent than carbohydrates and fats. When an individual is glycogen-depleted, she will burn more protein as fuel. It is not good to deplete the body of its essential protein; protein has numerous and vital roles in the human body outside of energy production, and should not be used as the major fuel source. So do not aim to burn protein as part of your exercise goals.

Even though the protein needs increase for those who are physically active, a balanced diet will definitely ensure an adequate intake. The recommendation for the protein requirement of the exercising female is 15 percent of total energy intake. This amount can easily be met through a balanced vegetarian/vegan diet. Soyfoods, nuts, and beans are excellent sources of protein.

Vitamins and Minerals

Vitamins and minerals play crucial roles in breaking down carbohydrates, proteins, and fats for fuel. They are also important in maintaining proper muscle function. Since physical activity increases the need for energy, the requirements for certain vitamins and minerals—such as the B-complex vitamins, which are essential for the production of energy—also increase.

Too many athletes feel that it is necessary to take large amounts of vitamin and mineral supplements in order to meet their nutritional requirements. There is no scientific research that indicates the enhancement of physical performance due to megadoses of vitamins and minerals. A well-balanced diet that provides nutrient-dense foods and a good multivitamin/mineral should adequately meet any additional vitamin and mineral needs that the physically active vegetarian female may have.

One nutrient that should be of special concern to physically active women is iron. Both male and female athletes are prone to iron depletion, though it does not seem to affect their performance directly. If the condition of iron depletion progresses to iron deficiency, physical performance *is* affected negatively. Iron deficiency anemia that is associated with athletes is frequently termed *runner's anemia* because it develops in many high-mileage runners. A deficiency of iron can lead to an inadequate supply of oxygen to the cells, which can be evidenced by easily becoming out of breath. Other symptoms are: pica (the craving of nonfoods, such as dirt, starch, clay, and ice); loss of stamina; inability to regulate body temperature; and reduced resistance to infections. It is vitally important that females who engage in regular physical activity have themselves screened periodically to assess iron status. Individuals who are assessed to have iron deficiency anemia will need iron supplementation therapy; they should follow the recommendations given by their doctors.

Sports anemia is different from true iron deficiency or runner's anemia. This condition is a temporary low hemoglobin concentration caused by a sudden increase in aerobic activity. It usually corrects itself after a few weeks of training and iron supplementation therapy is not required.

DAILY MEAL PATTERN GUIDELINES FOR THE PHYSICALLY ACTIVE VEGAN FEMALE

Refer to the meal pattern guide in Chapter 4, on page 47. If your calories and protein needs are closer to 40 to 50 grams of protein and 1,800 calories, focus on the lower half of the ranges. If your protein and calorie needs are higher, focus on the upper end of the ranges.

For the majority of women who exercise strenuously, regular iron supplementation is recommended; it is important to consult with a health-care professional on this matter. All women who exercise on a regular basis should strive to obtain at least 15 to 20 milligrams of iron per day, primarily through their diet, and through supplements if necessary. Iron-rich foods such as legumes, as well as vitamin C-rich foods, which enhance iron absorption, should be incorporated into the daily diet. See Table A.5 on page 240 for a list of iron-rich foods, and Table A.9 on page 243 for a list of vitamin C-rich foods.

Table 8.1 is a sample daily menu for the physically active vegan. You will notice that it offers a nice variety of foods that are both satisfying and healthy.

THE ADOLESCENT ATHLETE

Countless parents, coaches, and adolescent athletes are skeptical when it comes to a vegetarian diet. It's good to be skeptical—it shows that you are thinking hard about your health. But it is just as important to find the answers to your questions. The adolescent athlete can fully meet her nutritional needs on a vegetarian/vegan diet. Of course, as with any other athlete, she needs to plan her diet carefully so that it will support her activity.

Be assured that a vegan diet is able to supply all of the good quality protein that an adolescent athlete requires through legumes and grain. No protein supplements are needed, especially since protein is not the major source of fuel during exercise. We obtain most of our energy from carbohydrates. Therefore, the athletic adolescent vegetarian female should be sure to follow a high-carbohydrate diet.

It is crucial for the adolescent female who exercises to monitor her iron status regularly and to consume rich sources of iron daily. Her body is

Table 8.1. Sample Menu

Breakfast	Lunch	Dinner
1 whole wheat bagel	2 small whole wheat burrito shells	1 cup spinach brown rice
½ cup cream of wheat	1 cup stir-fried tofu (fajita style)	½ cup black-eye peas
1 cup fruit salad	1 cup lentil soup with ½ cup collards	½ cup butternut squash
1 cup fortified soymilk/soy beverage	2 fruits	1 cup raw vegetable salad
½ cup fortified orange juice	2 vegan cookies	1 tbsp salad dressing
	4 oz fruit juice	1 piece homemade cornbread
		4 oz vegetable juice

adjusting both to menstruation and to intense physical exertion. See page 240 for a list of iron-rich vegan foods. Iron supplementation is warranted a necessity for the adolescent with low iron status, but a physician must supervise it.

Eating disorders in young female athletes have become an epidemic problem that cannot be ignored. Some reports estimate that up to 62 percent of young athletes have been reported to engage in disordered eating, which includes both bulimia and anorexia nervosa. The adolescent who is driven to excel in her particular sport and who is pressured to fit a specific athletic image is certainly under a lot of pressure, and many turn to disordered eating to further increase control over their bodies. Christy Henrich is a sad example of the costly results of eating disorders. This 4'10" gymnast died at the tender age of 22, weighing only 65 pounds. It is important to realize that disordered eating is not an avenue of better control over your body. It does just the opposite—the eating disorder ends up controlling you.

THE DANGEROUS FEMALE ATHLETE TRIAD

The *female athlete triad* refers to the inter-relatedness of disordered eating, amenorrhea, and osteoporosis. This triad can lead to poor health and even death. First, diet is a constant concern for those who are physically active. A survey reported in the June 1992 edition of *Runners World* interviewed 4,500 females at an average age of 30 who trained seven to eight hours per week. Twenty-nine percent were dieting during periods of peak training; 48 percent were terrified of being overweight; 50 percent were preoccupied with a desire to be thin; 43 percent claimed they were out of control with their eating; 39 percent binged once a month or more; and 26 percent purged by using laxatives or diuretics. Obviously, disordered eating is a significant problem among the female athletic population.

Problems with the menstrual cycle can certainly be caused by improper or insufficient diet. The activities that require low body weight for aesthetic and competitive reasons—in such sports, for example, as ballet, gymnastics, and running—are associated with the highest incidence of menstrual dysfunction. *Athletic amenorrhea* (absence of menstruation) is the result of severe weight loss regimens and the strenuous exercise training programs that are common for many athletes. It has been shown to be associated with an increase in bone loss or lower bone density. These changes in bone health can result in more stress fractures and possibly osteoporosis in later life. Amenorrhea can also cause infertility. If athletic amenorrhea occurs, it is very important to adjust the diet and/or the exercise regimen.

A few studies—such as one published in 1984 by Slavin and colleagues, and another published in 1987 by Bruemmer and Drinkwater—have suggested that vegetarianism plays a role in athletic amenorrhea. The former study found that there was a higher percentage of amenorrhea in vegetarians in comparison to meat-eaters. This was most likely due largely (but not exclusively) to lower fat intake, which has an effect on menstrual function; compared with women who eat meat, vegetarian women have been found to have a lower percentage of body fat. Yet, fat can be added to a diet without the consumption of meat. And keep in mind that athletic amenorrhea is truly caused by multiple factors: diet; body composition; training regimen; reproductive maturity; and emotional and physical stress. It would be inaccurate to blame amenorrhea in vegetarian women on the fact that they do not consume flesh foods.

PRE- AND POST-COMPETITION TIPS

If you are an athlete who competes, you are most likely concerned with pre- and post-competition meals. You want to eat foods that make you feel energized and complete. Some tips for these critical times in an active female's athletic career are given below.

Pre-Competition Meal

The nutritional goal for the pre-competition meal is a high carbohydrate intake; usually, 55 to 70 percent of the total calories should come from this source. The carbohydrate foods should be high in starch—pastas, breads, potatoes, and rice are examples. Foods that are high in fiber, like raw fruits and vegetables with seeds and tough skin, are not recommended because they can cause intestinal discomfort. It is also recommended that you do *not* get your carbohydrates from simple sugars—for example, table sugar, brown sugar, honey, molasses, or products that contain these sweeteners, such as jellies, jams, and desserts. Simple sugars can cause a rapid rise in blood glucose and an overabundance of insulin, which ultimately can result in a low blood-glucose level and a feeling of tiredness.

Post-Competition Meal

It is within the first two hours after exercise that the muscles are most receptive to replacing muscle glycogen. Neglecting to consume adequate carbohydrates at this time can hinder optimal glycogen recovery and endurance. As a result, a serious deficit in stored glycogen can occur, especially for athletes who train regularly. In order to maximize the repletion process, 100 grams of carbohydrate should be consumed every two hours, for at least six hours. To help you gage this amount, one bagel has 30 grams of carbohydrate, a banana has 26.7 grams, and a cup of orange juice has 26.8 grams.

Fluid Requirements

To remain hydrated before, during, and after exercise or competition, drink large amounts of fluids. Two hours before exertion, drink approximately 2 cups of fluid. Then, another 2 cups should be consumed every fifteen to twenty minutes during exertion.

The amount of fluid to drink after competition should be based on the number of pounds lost. For every pound of weight lost during competition, a pint of water should be consumed. Water is the best fluid replacer. However, exercise in excess of one hour and/or exercise in extreme environmental conditions, such as high temperature and high humidity, may require the consumption of sports beverages. These drinks contain essential electrolytes and carbohydrates.

The importance of exercise as a part of a healthy lifestyle cannot be overestimated. Exercise agendas should not be looked upon as added burdens to our lives. Instead, we need to view them as wise and profitable investments, much like healthy eating. The more energy and time that we give to our physical activity, the more we get out of it.

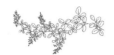 # Chapter 9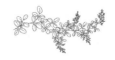

The Pregnant
and the Breastfeeding
Vegetarian

Odessa and George Primer were expecting their fourth child. Odessa had delivered three healthy babies in the past. Yet, she was a bit nervous because her family recently decided to become vegans. When Odessa told her doctor about her dietary decision, he immediately stated that she was putting herself and her child in a dangerous situation. He strongly advised her to see a dietitian because he felt she was at "high nutritional risk."

Odessa sought the advice of a dietitian who also followed a vegan diet. As soon as the visit began, Odessa's fears were put to rest. The dietitian not only gave Odessa a number of resources to read, such as "The Vegetarian Mother and Baby Book" by Rose Elliot, but she even made a sample diet plan for Odessa to follow. Today, daughter Chawnice is a healthy, active, and intelligent 9-year-old, and Odessa and George are proud they stuck with their dietary convictions. Odessa's story illustrates that a female can receive full nutritional support from a plant-based diet, even during times of the greatest nutritional demands.

The pregnant vegetarian—and any pregnant woman, for all that matters—must eat the best foods in order to adequately nourish herself and the fetus who is growing inside of her. Similarly, during lactation, the mother not only has to feed herself well, but also must produce healthy food for her infant. Unfortunately, many health professionals do not study the vegetarian diet and, therefore, express disapproval of following vegetarianism throughout pregnancy and lactation. Can a vegetarian diet nutritionally support the female during these life stages? This chapter will address that question. Hopefully, by the end, you will feel confident that, as a vegetarian, you can provide optimal nutrition for both yourself and your child.

PREGNANCY AND NUTRITION

Pregnancy should be a time of joy and great expectancy. In addition, it should be a time during which the woman takes a special interest in her eating and lifestyle habits. So much of who that baby will be depends upon the decisions the mother makes while the baby is still within her womb. Malnutrition in women prior to pregnancy and throughout pregnancy is associated with: miscarriages; stillbirths; premature births; and infants who suffer from low birth weight, neural tube defects, congenital malformations, and mental and physical retardation. So, from the moment of conception to the birth of the baby and beyond, nutrition is vital.

Essential Vitamins and Minerals

In order for the baby to develop properly, the mother must ingest more nutrients than when she wasn't pregnant. Certain nutrients are especially important, while the requirements for others do not change. Table 9.1 on page 97 highlights several daily nutrient requirements for women before pregnancy, followed by requirements during pregnancy. *These are minimum requirements; you may require greater amounts according to your individual needs.* Some of these nutrients warrent further discussion.

Calcium

In Table 9.1, you will note that there is no increase in calcium requirements when a female becomes pregnant. However, too many women do not meet their daily requirement as it is, and an adequate intake of calcium is especially important during the last two trimesters of pregnancy (that is, the last six months). That's when the bones of the fetus are developing. For a list of calcium-rich vegan food sources, see Table A.2 on page 236. Your obstetrician will also suggest various methods of calcium supplementation.

Folate (Folic Acid)

Folate has received much media attention because of its confirmed influence on birth defects. *Spina bifida* is a neural tube defect in which the spinal column of the infant does not completely close. It usually results in varying degrees of paralysis. Every year, 1,500 to 3,000 children in the United States are affected by spina bifida. Numerous studies have concluded not only that this birth defect is preventable, but also that folate is responsible for prevention.

Table 9.1. Comparison of Daily Nutrient Requirements Prior to Pregnancy and During Pregnancy				
Nutrient	Requirement During Childbearing Years		Requirement During Pregnancy	
	14–18 years	19–50 years	14–18 years	19–50 years
Calcium	1,300 mg	1,000 mg	1,300 mg	1,000 mg
Folate (Folic Acid)	400 mcg	400 mcg	600 mcg	600 mcg
Iron	15 mg	15 mg	30 mg	30 mg
Magnesium	360 mg	310–320 mg	400 mg	350–360 mg
Pantothenic Acid	5 mg	5 mg	6 mg	6 mg
Vitamin B_1 (Thiamin)	1.0 mg	1.1 mg	1.4 mg	1.4 mg
Vitamin B_2 (Riboflavin)	1.0 mg	1.1 mg	1.4 mg	1.4 mg
Vitamin B_3 (Niacin)	14 mg	14 mg	18 mg	18 mg
Vitamin B_6 (Pyridoxine)	1.2 mg	1.3 mg	1.9 mg	1.9 mg
Vitamin B_{12} (Cobalamin)	2.4 mcg	2.4 mcg	2.6 mcg	2.6 mcg
Vitamin D	5 mcg	5 mcg	5 mcg	5 mcg
Zinc	12 mg	12 mg	15 mg	15 mg

However, ensuring an adequate folate consumption once a female knows that she is pregnant will not prevent this devastating disorder. *The nutrient must be taken in adequate amounts before pregnancy and during the early development of the embryo.* Most females do not even know they are pregnant for the first couple of weeks. This means that women in their childbearing years must make sure they are consuming adequate daily amounts of folate.

A vegetarian who is consuming a balanced diet will certainly obtain sufficient amounts of folate because vegan foods are the richest source of this nutrient. One cup of lentils provides practically two-thirds of the daily requirement of folate for the pregnant female. See Table A.4 on page 239 for a list of folate-rich vegan foods.

Iron

A pregnant woman needs to absorb more iron than her body loses. The growth of the fetus and the placenta that nourishes it requires increased numbers of red blood cells and, thus, more iron. Pregnancy is associated with a heightened risk for iron deficiency.

Often, diets low in *both* meat and vitamin C (ascorbic acid) are considered risk factors for iron deficiency. As discussed in Chapter 5, red meat provides heme iron, which the body easily absorbs, while vitamin C enhances iron absorption. Obviously, the vegetarian diet contains no meat, but by no means should it also be low in vitamin C. In fact, just the opposite is characteristic of a well-balanced vegetarian diet; it is extremely high in vitamin C, since it emphasizes fruits and vegetables that are rich in this nutrient.

Pregnant vegetarian females need to take special note concerning the importance of vitamin C for iron absorption. A vitamin C-rich drink like orange juice can double the amount of iron absorbed from a plant-based meal. Meanwhile, milk, tea, or coffee can cut the absorption of iron from plant foods by more than half.

Due to the increased demand for blood during pregnancy, and to the loss of blood at delivery, the iron requirements for pregnant females double. (See Table 9.1, page 97.) It is difficult to meet the high recommended levels of iron from diet alone. Thus, supplements should be taken. *Be sure to take iron supplements as prescribed by your obstetrician.* Usually, the prenatal vitamin manages this requirement.

To further increase iron intake and absorption during pregnancy, purchase a cast-iron skillet. The food that you cook in the skillet will absorb iron and you will benefit from this extra source. And again, eat vitamin C-rich foods with iron-rich foods, because ascorbic acid enhances the absorption of iron. For a list of iron-rich vegan foods, see Table A.5 on page 241. For a list of vitamin C-rich foods, see Table A.9 on page 243.

Vitamin B_{12}

Because it is found almost exclusively in animal foods, vitamin B_{12} is a concern, especially for vegans. However, there are only a few recorded incidences of vitamin-B_{12} deficiency in infants of vegan mothers. These infants were breastfed, and so vitamin B_{12} will be discussed under "Breastfeeding, Nutrition, and the Vegetarian Diet," on page 103. Please refer to page 243 for reliable vegan sources of vitamin B_{12}. If a reliable source is not being consumed, supplementation is necessary.

Vitamin D

Vitamin D is also of special concern during pregnancy; it is an important nutrient in the fetus' proper bone formation. Vitamin D increases the absorption of calcium from the gastrointestinal tract. Thus, the pregnant vegan should make efforts to consume foods that are fortified with this nutrient. See page 244 for a list of several such products. To enhance intake even further, the pregnant female should receive adequate daily sunlight and take a supplement that contains vitamin D.

Zinc

Zinc takes part in the production of genetic material—DNA and RNA. Adequate amounts are essential during pregnancy. Zinc deficiency, though rarely reported in pregnant females, has been associated with neural tube defects, congenital malformations, and pregnancy and delivery complications. Please refer to Table A.11 on page 244 for a list of zinc-rich vegan foods, and be sure that if you are pregnant, you increase your zinc intake.

Weight Changes

Pregnancy naturally means weight gain, and the vegan diet can provide the necessary nutrients to promote it. Weight gain becomes a critical issue during pregnancy because the pre-pregnancy weight of the female compared with her weight gain (amount and progression) during pregnancy is two of the main indicators of the nutritional status of the mother and the growing fetus. A pre-pregnancy weight that is more than 10 percent under, or more than 20 percent over, a woman's ideal body weight places her at greater risk

A Word About Prenatal Vitamins

Prenatal supplements are strongly recommended for the vegan/vegetarian pregnant woman, to ensure a reliable source of nutrients. The case of iron, alone, makes a strong argument for supplementation; the increased demands during pregnancy and the loss of blood during childbirth necessitate that the mother builds her iron stores throughout the pregnancy. While most pregnant moms strive for an optimal dietary nutrition intake during this time, the nutrient goals may not be reached every day, and a prenatal supplement can supply the need when the diet is lacking. *Nature's Plus High Potency Ultra Prenatal, Rainbow Light Complete Prenatal System, Schiff New Beginning Prenatal,* and *Solgar's Prenatal Nutrients* are recommended vegetarian/vegan prenatal supplements.

for complications during pregnancy. In addition, the chance of a low-birth-weight infant increases if the woman is underweight before pregnancy.

Recent statistics and current recommendations for weight gain in pregnant females propose that a total of 25 to 30 pounds should be gained during pregnancy, if the female was at a healthy pre-pregnancy weight. This weight gain should occur gradually throughout the pregnancy. During the first trimester (the first three months), approximately 3 pounds should be gained. Then, about 1 pound should be gained every week throughout the second and third trimesters. However, a female who was underweight at the time of her baby's conception needs to add more pounds throughout gestation; 28 to 40 pounds is recommended. And the overweight female does not need to gain as much during pregnancy; the recommendation is 15 to 25 pounds. Of course, a woman pregnant with twins needs to gain more weight—35 to 45 pounds. Other multiple birth situations require additional weight gain.

Just as you need to get rid of 3,500 calories to lose a pound of weight, you need to consume an additional 3,500 calories to put on a pound of weight. This amounts to approximately 500 additional calories a day in order to gain a pound per week. The RDA for pregnant women recommends an additional 300 calories per day instead, especially since only 3 pounds of weight gain is suggested for the first trimester. A pregnant female must also consume additional protein. The Recommended Dietary Allowance (RDA) suggests an additional 10 grams of protein per day.

So the pregnant female has to consume more vitamins and minerals, more calories, and more protein. Exactly how is the vegetarian, and moreover the vegan diet supposed to accomplish this amazing feat? When we talk about foods that help us to gain weight, we often think of meat, milk, and dairy products, and the numerous foods that contain these ingredients. In health-care facilities, a traditional way to help patients gain weight is to give them whole-milk, custards and puddings, cream, butter/margarine on bread, and milk shakes. We hardly ever see vegan foods, except for nuts and avocados, that appear on these lists. But is it possible to increase your weight on plant foods?

Nutrient-dense foods are the magic words that will enable the pregnant vegetarian/vegan to support the growth of her unborn child, as well as her own health. They will help her boost her calories and protein intake and will supply the essential nutrients. Among the best types of foods that can live up to this high standard are nuts and seeds. They are simply packed with calories, protein, and nutrients. For example, 1 cup of almonds provides 837 calories; 28 grams of protein; 378 milligrams of calcium; 5.2 milligrams of iron; and 83 micrograms of folate. An additional $\frac{1}{2}$ cup of nuts a day will give the pregnant female most of the extra nutrients her body needs. Other non-animal food products that can increase the intake of calories, protein, vitamins, and minerals are listed in Table 9.2.

In addition to the foods listed below, increasing portion sizes and drinking fruit and vegetable juices will help to provide the extra nutrition needed during pregnancy. It is not difficult to gain weight on a vegan diet. Remember, though, that chowing down on potato chips and *Top Ramen* is not the way to go. High-fat foods, especially foods that are high in saturated fats and contain little or no essential nutrients, will result in excessive weight gain, while increasing your risk of conditions such as heart disease. Also, they will add to establishing poor eating habits, which can lead to nutritional deficiencies, especially during pregnancy and lactation.

Daily Meal Pattern Guidelines for the Pregnant Vegan

Please refer to the meal pattern guide in Chapter 4, page 47, for a basic outline of food groups and serving numbers. There are few adjustments to

Table 9.2. Power-Packed Vegan Foods					
Food	**Serving Size**	**Calories**	**Protein (g)**	**Calcium (mg)**	**Iron (mg)**
Blackstrap molasses	2 tbsp	94	–	344	7.00
Brewer's yeast	1 oz	80	11.0	60	4.90
Figs, dried	10 each	477	5.7	269	4.18
Granola, homemade	$\frac{1}{4}$ cup	138	3.5	18	1.13
Natto	$\frac{1}{2}$ cup	187	15.6	191	7.57
Nutbutters	1 tbsp	95	4.0	30	1.00
Nuts	1 oz	165	5.5	57	1.70
Soybeans	1 cup	298	28.6	175	8.84
Soynuts	$\frac{1}{4}$ cup	194	17.0	116	1.70
Tempeh	$\frac{1}{2}$ cup	165	15.7	77	1.88
Tofu pudding	1 cup	250	18.0	80	2.70
Tortula yeast	1 oz	79	10.9	120	5.50
Wheat germ, toasted	$\frac{1}{4}$ cup	108	8.0	13	2.60

make if you are pregnant. Most pregnant females will need to increase servings from the starch, legumes, nuts, and tofu (soy products) food groups by one serving per day. Also, one to two servings of foods containing more than 200 milligrams of calcium, such as calcium-fortified orange juice and soymilk/soy drink, are strongly recommended to ensure an adequate calcium intake.

The menu offered in Table 9.3 suggests three balanced meals in accordance with the meal pattern described above. From the food choices listed below, you can see that the healthy vegan mom-to-be can enjoy lots of flavor, texture, and variety.

Support for Veganism

After reading this chapter thus far, you should feel confident that a vegan diet can support the needs of the pregnant female, as long as careful consideration and time are taken to ensure an adequate intake of all the necessary nutrients. In order to do this, a balanced diet and nutritional supplements are necessary. However, if you'd feel better knowing that research studies have supported veganism and confidently published the results, a few examples of such studies are worth discussing.

J. Thomas and F.R. Ellis performed a study in which they looked at the health of vegans during pregnancy. The results of their research showed that the vegan diet did not have any adverse effects on the mothers or the children during pregnancy. Furthermore, when compared with meat-eaters, the vegan group had a lower incidence of toxemia (blood poisoning) of pregnancy. There were no significant differences between the vegans and the omnivores concerning the occurrence of miscarriages or of anemia during pregnancy.

Table 9.3. Sample Menu

Breakfast	Lunch	Dinner
$\frac{1}{2}$ cup granola	2 vegan tacos made with vegan burgers	1 cup *Tuno*, spinach, macaroni casserole (pkg)
1 cup fortified soymilk	1 cup carrot sticks	
1 oatbran English muffin	5 dried figs	$\frac{1}{2}$ cup seasoned soybeans
$\frac{1}{2}$ cup scrambled tofu	$\frac{1}{4}$ cup nuts	$\frac{1}{2}$ cup carrots
1 cup sliced banana and strawberries	1 cup calcium-fortified orange juice	Small tossed salad with raw broccoli florets
2 tbsp wheat germ		1 cup peach nectar

So rest assured that if you have chosen vegetarianism or veganism, you are not going to harm your unborn child or yourself by sticking to your convictions. In fact, you are taking a healthy step toward optimal nutrition.

Carter and colleagues also performed studies looking at pregnant vegan females. These studies were conducted at "The Farm," a vegetarian community in Tennessee. They concluded that women who adhere to a vegan diet are able to achieve normal and healthy pregnancies with appropriate prenatal care and a well-balanced vegan diet that includes prenatal supplements. In addition, after reviewing the record of 775 vegan mothers, the researchers concluded that the vegan diet could alleviate most if not all symptoms of *preeclampsia*—a medical problem in pregnancy associated with increasing high blood pressure, edema (swelling), protein in the urine, and possible convulsions. It has been theorized that the cause of preeclampsia is nutrition related.

BREASTFEEDING, NUTRITION, AND THE VEGETARIAN DIET

Once you've completed the pregnancy stage and given birth to your infant, lactation begins. Lactation—the secretion of milk from the mammary glands—places extra nutritional demands on the body. But breastfeeding is the most natural and nutritious way to provide for an infant's dietary requirements. It supplies all of the nutrients that the infant needs and is naturally structured for easy digestion. Breastfeeding also emotionally and socially nourishes your baby. Yes, breastmilk is the most perfect food for your child, just as cow's milk is the most perfect food for the baby calf. The American Pediatric Association states, "Exclusive breast-feeding is the preferred method of feeding for normal full-term infants from birth to 6 months."

The advantages of breastfeeding are plentiful. In addition to those discussed above, breastmilk—particularly over the first few days after birth—strengthens the child's immunity in ways that manufactured infant formulas cannot. Also, it is the most economical way to feed your child. Eating an additional 500 calories daily in food to supplement for the extra demands that lactation makes on your body will cost you significantly less than the daily cost of formula.

The study conducted by Ellis and Thomas, mentioned on page 102, revealed an extremely positive trait in vegan mothers; researchers found that the vegan mothers were more likely than meat-eaters to breastfeed their infants. This is an exciting trend for the vegetarian female population. It goes to show that women who choose not to consume animal products are extending their health interests to other areas of their lives (and their children's lives).

If the mother is consuming a healthy and balanced diet that is rich in all of the essential nutrients, her breastmilk, in turn, will be rich in all of the essential nutrients. (One exception is vitamin D; see page 105.) The mother actually produces more milk during the first six months of breastfeeding than the following six months. This makes perfect sense; as the infant begins to consume more solid food and less milk, the mother's body adjusts. Mothers who choose not to breastfeed their infants put their bodies through a rapid and often painful transition.

Essential Vitamins and Minerals

If a mother's diet is lacking in essential nutrients, specifically the water-soluble nutrients, the breastfed infant's diet may also be lacking in these nutrients. Water-soluble vitamins, such as vitamins B_6 and C, must be replenished daily. Quite differently, fat-soluble vitamins, such as vitamins A and E, are able to be stored in the body for long periods of time. Therefore, you can pull from these stores when you need extra. Table 9.4 lists the nutrients that are required in greater demand during lactation and, for each one, offers a comparison of required amounts during pre-pregnancy and lactation. *The figures in the table are minimum requirements; you may need greater amounts of specific nutrients, according to your specific needs.*

Table 9.4. Changes in Nutrient Requirements From Pre-Pregnancy to Lactation		
	Pre-Pregnancy Requirement		Requirement During
Nutrient	14–18 years	19–50 years	Lactation
Biotin	25 mg	30 mg	35 mg
Folate (Folic Acid)	400 mcg	400 mcg	500 mcg
Pantothenic Acid	5 mg	5 mg	7 mg
Vitamin B_1 (Thiamin)	1.0 mg	1.1 mg	1.5 mg
Vitamin B_2 (Riboflavin)	1.0 mg	1.1 mg	1.6 mg
Vitamin B_3 (Niacin)	14 mg	14 mg	17 mg
Vitamin B_6 (Pyridoxine)	1.2 mg	1.3 mg	2.0 mg
Vitamin B_{12} (Cobalamin)	2.4 mcg	2.4 mcg	2.8 mcg

Vitamins B_{12} and D are both stored in the body for long periods of time. The first is water soluble, while the second is fat soluble. The requirement for vitamin D does not change during lactation, while the necessary increase in vitamin B_{12} is listed in Table 9.4, above. A woman who is not getting adequate amounts of these nutrients in her diet will have small stores, if any. This places both her and especially her infant at risk of vitamin deficiency.

Vitamin B_{12}

Vitamin B_{12} intake is a special point of interest for vegans. The words *veganism* and *lactation* are usually found with the term *vitamin-B_{12} deficiency*. Most health-care professionals, including dietitians, often point to this triad as a case against veganism, especially during pregnancy and lactation. However, the belief that a vegan mother breastfeeding her child will most likely lead to vitamin-B_{12} deficiency in the child is based only on a few case studies. Careful research of medical literature reveals that vitamin-B_{12} deficiency in vegans is the exception to the rule. Furthermore, in cases in which deficiency was reported, there is some question as to whether it was truly caused solely by a lack of vitamin B_{12} in the diet.

Researchers have yet to figure out why many infants of vegan mothers do not develop a vitamin-B_{12} deficiency, though there are several theories. In the meantime, pregnant and lactating vegans should make sure that they are receiving an adequate supply of this nutrient from reliably fortified sources. See page 243 for a list of such products.

Vitamin D

The necessary amount of vitamin D cannot adequately be provided by non-fortified foods. Vitamin D can be obtained through fortified products, sunlight, and pill supplementation. Be sure to take 400 IU daily.

Calorie and Protein Requirements

Breastfeeding actually increases a female's nutritional requirements for energy and protein more than pregnancy does. This is because the female body must not only replace its depleted stores immediately after the birth of the infant, but also must produce nutritious milk. Breastfeeding increases the mother's energy needs to an additional 500 calories per day. An additional 15 grams of protein need to be consumed daily during the first six months of breastfeeding, while the following six months require 12 grams over the nonpregnant, nonlactating requirement.

Fluid Requirements

The breastfeeding mother must also increase her fluid intake. She should drink at least six to eight (8-ounce) glasses of water every day. *In addition*, copious amounts of fruit/vegetable juices and soymilk or nut milk should be included in the diet.

Many health professionals make the mistake of thinking that milk is an essential part of the lactating mother's diet. They advise the mother to increase her milk intake during this stage. Please know that it is only a false myth that you must drink milk in order to lactate. The hormone *prolactin,* which triggers milk production in the breast, is naturally produced in the pregnant and lactating female and has nothing to do with the ingestion of dairy products. So even if you are a vegan, you need not doubt your dietary convictions. Vegan foods are able to provide all of the nutrients required for lactation, and such foods do not contain some of the questionable substances found in cow's milk, such as hormones.

Chapter 2 discusses pesticides such as PDB, PCB, DDT, and DDE in the food supply. Dairy cows ingest these toxins in large amounts, and the chemicals are retained in the fat in the animals' bodies. When women, in particular, eat the flesh or drink the milk of animals that contain these compounds, the substances are also retained in the women's bodies, specifically in the breasts and other areas that are composed largely of fat. When the mother breastfeeds her baby, what do you think happens? Exactly! The infant receives these compounds in the breastmilk, thus being placed at risk of experiencing harmful effects. For a list of other substances that may contaminate breastmilk, see "Contaminated Breastmilk" on page 107.

Daily Meal Pattern Guidelines for the Lactating Vegan

Refer to the meal pattern guide in Chapter 4, on page 47, and make the following adjustments. A breastfeeding mom should add one to two extra servings from the whole grains, legumes, tofu, or nuts/seeds groups. In addition, as mentioned previously, she should be absolutely sure to consume at least six to eight (8-ounce) glasses of water every day, plus juices and nondairy "milks." Calcium-fortified orange juice and soymilk/soy drinks should be included in this fluid intake.

THE PREGNANT AND LACTATING TEEN

Though the timing of growth and sexual maturation differs for each female, adolescent females generally reach physiological maturity approximately four years after their first menstruation. A pregnancy prior to the end of

---

Contaminated Breastmilk

Chemicals and hormones that are ingested by food animals certainly enter the bodies of the people who consume the animals' flesh and milk. These substances can be passed to breastfeeding infants. In addition to meat and dairy products, there are other substances that can contaminate breastmilk and negatively affect our children, including alcohol, cocaine and other illegal drugs, and certain medications such as *Tagamet* (used in the treatment of ulcers, heartburn, and esophagitis) and *Tavist* (an antihistamine). For the sake of your baby, it is important to do the right thing: completely avoid these substances during pregnancy and lactation. If you have any questions regarding the effect of a food, beverage, or medication on your breastmilk, consult a health-care professional.

---

these four years presents health concerns for the growing teenager. Pregnant teenagers simultaneously face two critical times in the life cycle of a female—adolescence and pregnancy. Both of these times are characterized by growth, development, and heightened nutritional needs.

A Time for Heightened Awareness

The infant mortality rate is high for mothers under the age of twenty, and it's even higher for mothers under the age of fifteen. That's not to say that there's only a small chance of infant survival if the mother is very young. Her body is very capable of gestation, delivery, and lactation. It just means that the pregnant adolescent must be extremely attentive to the multiple challenges that her growing body is experiencing. If she is informed, her chances for a healthy baby are wonderful.

Daily Meal Pattern Guidelines for the Pregnant and the Lactating Adolescent Vegan

Refer to the meal pattern guide in Chapter 4, page 47. The pregnant or lactating adolescent should consume the mid to upper range of the servings per day. It is vital that she choose the richest sources of nutrients from each food group, and that she take prenatal vitamins (see the inset on page 99). As previously mentioned, calcium-fortified orange juice and soymilk/soy drinks are strongly recommended. To ensure an adequate intake weekly, menus should be prepared ahead of time.

Both pregnancy and breastfeeding increase a female's nutrient requirements. I hope this chapter has given you confidence in how nutrient-dense vegan foods, fortified foods, and supplements (as directed by your physician) are able to fully provide for the female's and the growing baby's nutritional needs. In fact, considering that a plant-based diet will also reduce the risk—both child's and mother's—of foodborne illnesses and exposure to chemicals and hormones pumped into food animals, a vegan diet seems safer and smarter.

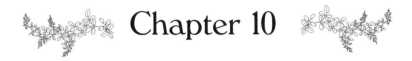

Chapter 10

The Vegetarian Senior

Sylvia Slater is very active and pleasant at 80 years of age. She has enjoyed a life free from disease and illness. Mrs. Slater raised three children and two grandchildren, and is now helping to raise her granddaughter's child. She is active in her church and loves to help other seniors who are not faring as well. Sylvia also enjoys a brisk walk around her neighborhood every morning; it keeps her feeling vibrant.

Sylvia believes her great health is a direct result of a lifestyle that includes: a strong devotional life; daily exercise; the avoidance of alcohol, drugs, and caffeine; and eating vegan. Sylvia has been a vegetarian for sixty-three years. She was a lacto-ovovegetarian for a long time and, in 1969, decided to go all the way. Sylvia has been a vegan—and an extremely healthy woman—ever since.

Statistics have shown that the number of people living past the age of 65 has been continuously, even drastically, increasing in the United States and throughout the world. It is important to obtain a better knowledge and understanding of the nutritional requirements particular to this population group, especially because you are either in it or are heading that way. This chapter will discuss the nutritional requirements of seniors and how they can be fulfilled through a vegetarian diet.

COMMON SENIOR HEALTH CONCERNS AND THE VEGETARIAN DIET

Fear and anxiety are two of the many feelings that we may experience when we think of growing older. That is because many of us associate aging with disease. Unfortunately, aging does involve the gradual deterioration of many systems in the human body, and this leads to certain disabilities. Yet, few people actually die of old age. Many seniors suffer and die from debilitating diseases that could have been prevented.

For example, countless incidences of heart disease and cancer—the major causes of death in the United States—could have been prevented by better lifestyle habits. In addition, diabetes and osteoporosis are often the results of a lifetime of poor choices. The risk for all of these diseases increases significantly as we age, so seniors need to make special efforts to inform themselves about nutrition.

Becoming a senior citizen can and should be characterized by good health achieved through proper eating habits, regular exercise, and a happy emotional status. Even if a disease does exist, establishing good health habits may improve and, in some cases, reverse the disease process. As at any point in the life cycle, nutrition plays a major role in determining whether a person will suffer from debilitating chronic diseases or will enjoy the blessings of good health. Balanced vegetarian eating promotes health and vitality in the senior body.

Nieman and associates conducted a study, published in the *Journal of the American Dietetic Association* in 1989, that involved thirty-seven women aged 65 to 80 years. Twenty-three of the women were vegetarians and fourteen were omnivores. The purpose of the study was to determine and compare the nutrient intakes of the vegetarians with the nonvegetarians. The study concluded that the vegetarian women had nutrient profiles that corresponded more closely with the Recommended Dietary Allowances. They consumed more carbohydrates; more dietary fiber; more of seven vitamins and minerals; less saturated fat; less dietary cholesterol; and less caffeine. Based on all of these results, the study suggests that the vegetarian diet is a healthier and more nutritious diet than the omnivorous diet. It has the benefits with which seniors should be most concerned.

Preventing and Treating Chronic Disease

Vegetarianism is associated with lower risk of heart disease, high blood pressure, cancer, diabetes, and osteoporosis. Seniors are more concerned than anyone else is when it comes to such chronic disorders. It is important for seniors to realize that vegetarianism can help.

According to Suzanne Havala—a registered dietitian, primary author of the American Dietetic Association's position paper on vegetarian diets, and nutrition adviser for the Vegetarian Resource Group—vegetarian diets for seniors can help to control high blood pressure, heart disease, and other conditions. The Nieman study discussed on page 110 reported that female senior vegetarians consume a diet that is similar to the guidelines advocated by the American Heart Association and the National Cancer Institute. The researchers concluded that seniors benefit from the vegetarian diet because it ranks low in the promotion of heart disease and because it improves the intake levels of most nutrients. See Chapters 12 through 18 for specific details on how vegetarianism prevents and/or helps combat specific chronic diseases.

Preventing Arthritis

Arthritis is a disease that generally afflicts the elderly, and primarily occurs in females. There are many different kinds of arthritis. One common type is *rheumatoid arthritis,* a connective tissue disease that causes an often painful inflammation of the joints and usually affects several joints at once. Many people don't realize that animal fat can cause and/or worsen joint inflammation. Also, allergic reactions to meat—or the drugs, hormones, and chemicals in it—can manifest as the symptoms of arthritis. So avoiding meat can actually help your arthritis! Chapter 18 discusses rheumatoid arthritis in detail and explains research that has found vegetarianism to be beneficial in reducing the symptoms (see page 202).

Preventing Constipation

A condition that is prevalent among seniors, especially those residing in nursing homes, is constipation. Chronic constipation is defined as the difficult or infrequent passage of feces. In most cases, the first line of treatment includes a high-fiber diet. Fiber helps retain the health and tone of the intestinal muscles and attracts water to the intestinal tract, which softens the stool. Fruits, vegetables, and whole grains are excellent sources of fiber. Vegetarians have been found to consume more fiber than meat-eaters.

The current recommendation for fiber is 20 to 35 grams per day, which can easily be met on a vegan/vegetarian diet. The optimal dosage would be a daily intake of 35 grams or more. Instead of turning immediately to laxatives, try bran, prune juice, and dried fruit such as prunes or figs, as these vegan foods have a laxative effect. Adequate fluid consumption is also essential in the prevention and treatment of constipation.

Preventing Dementia

The vegetarian diet has been shown to have a trend towards delayed onset of dementia in the aged. In a study done by Giem and colleagues, the relationship between animal-product consumption and dementia was investigated in 272 individuals. The researchers found that individuals who consumed meat (including poultry and fish) in their diets were twice as likely to be afflicted with dementia than their vegetarian counterparts.

CHANGES IN NUTRIENT REQUIREMENTS

As individuals get older, energy needs decrease. Retirement, less physical activity, physical ailments, and a decreased metabolic rate are all factors that contribute to lower energy requirements. These decreased calorie needs make it mandatory that the food that is consumed by the senior is nutrient-dense.

Dietary surveys of older people in the United States have shown that this group is more likely to experience malnutrition than other population groups. A 20- to 25-percent decrease in caloric intake is associated with a decrease in the intake of vitamins and minerals as age progresses from 30 to 80 years. Though most of the vitamin and mineral recommendations do not change for women past the age of 50, there are four nutrient intakes that should be adjusted. As shown in Table 10.1, the requirements for vitamins B_6 and D, as well as for calcium, increase. Due to *menopause*—the ending of the menstrual flow—iron needs decrease. *Keep in mind that DRIs are adequate, but not necessarily optimal requirements; your individual case may require greater nutrient intakes.*

The study of gerontology, which focuses on the biology, psychology, and sociology of aging, began only recently. There is still much debate concerning the special nutrient needs of seniors. As the debate continues, older adults should be careful to obtain *at least* the current nutrient recommendations assigned by the Daily Reference Intakes (see Table A.1 on page 234). They can do this by following a well-balanced vegan diet that emphasizes nutrient-dense foods, fortified foods, and/or a daily multivitamin.

Table 10.1. Changes in Nutrient Intakes			
Nutrient	**DRI for Female, 31–50 years**	**DRI for Female, 50–71 years**	**DRI for Female, > 71 Years**
Calcium	1,000 mg	1,200 mg	1,200 mg
Iron	12.0 mg	10.0 mg	10.0 mg
Vitamin B_6	1.3 mg	1.5 mg	1.5 mg
Vitamin D	5 mcg	10 mcg	15 mcg

COMMON SENIOR PROBLEMS THAT RESULT IN POOR NUTRITION

There are several common problems that negatively affect the nutrition of many seniors. Loss of appetite, dehydration, and chewing difficulties are discussed below. If you or your loved one is experiencing any of these problems, be sure to take measures to remedy the situation so that optimal nutrient intake can be achieved.

Loss of Appetite

Loss of appetite and resulting poor dietary intake are very common among seniors. A major contributor to reduced appetite is depression, and it's frequently seen in the aged. Depression can occur for a number of reasons. Some of these are: the loss of a spouse or loved one; having to be admitted to an adult-care facility; reduced physical independence; and realization of changing mental processes. These traumatic and heart-breaking experiences can lead to feelings of loneliness that easily result in a lack of interest in food. The senior who is suffering from depression and/or loneliness and, in turn, poor nutrition should attempt to socialize with others. Participating in activities may begin to take her focus off her sorrows and onto the development of new relationships.

Using multiple medications at one time can also be the cause of loss of appetite. In addition, some drugs suppress the appetite or cause adverse responses to food—loss of taste, nausea, vomiting. If you suspect a particular drug to be the problem, talk with the physician to see if the prescription can be changed. If it cannot, try eating foods that have strong flavors. Such foods help to eliminate nausea or the urgency to vomit, and they are easier to taste.

Seniors experience a general decline in their sense of smell and taste. Both of these senses are essential in stimulating the desire to eat. Being able to smell freshly baked bread or onions and garlic simmering on the stove does a lot for awakening the appetite. Bland foods do not offer much to either smell or taste, but potent and strong flavored foods can help to improve the appetite.

Eating smaller and more frequent meals might also help, as smaller meals are less overwhelming. Also, preparing familiar and favorite foods might stimulate the appetite. Nutritional-supplement beverages provide an excellent source of concentrated calories and other nutrients when dietary intake is inadequate. However, few of these products are prepared with the vegan in mind. If you are vegan, preparing your own nutritionally-packed beverage is not difficult and can actually be much less expensive than purchasing commercially prepared products.

Dehydration

Older individuals may be at high risk of dehydration—the loss of too much fluid from the body. Dehydration occurs for a number of reasons, including: the inability to obtain water because of physical limitations; not paying attention to or responding to thirst, sometimes to avoid frequent trips to the bathroom; and simply not feeling thirsty. Two research studies found that vegetarian seniors were consuming inadequate amounts of fluid. Generally, 6 to 8 cups of fluid should be consumed daily by older adults. Juices are an alternative to water; they provide more taste, as well as some needed calories, vitamins, and minerals.

If you are not drinking at least six cups of fluid a day, photocopy the chart on page 255 and place it on your fridge as a reminder. This way, when you go into the kitchen, you will be motivated to get something to drink. Every time you drink a cup of fluid, put a check in the appropriate box. Another way to motivate yourself is to prepare delicious shakes and juices. See "Tofu Strawberry Shake," below, for a wonderful recipe.

Chewing Difficulties

A vegetarian diet can be a challenge for those who have oral problems such as missing teeth or ill-fitting dentures. Furthermore, some seniors prefer not to use dentures. Fresh fruit and vegetables, as well as certain whole

---

Tofu Strawberry Shake

Our bodies require a lot of fluid. In the hot weather, when risk of dehydration becomes even greater, we crave cold, refreshing drinks. Try a tofu strawberry shake for a healthy and tasty treat. It's easy to make.

> Half of a 12.3-oz package of *Mori Nu Tofu* (firm)
> $1\frac{1}{2}$ cups frozen strawberries (no sugar added)
> 1 cup *EdenSoy* soymilk
> $\frac{1}{3}$ cup sugar
> $\frac{1}{8}$ tsp vanilla extract

Blend all ingredients in a blender until smooth. This recipe yields two 8-ounce servings.

grains and nuts, can be difficult to chew and swallow.

Cooking—simmering, steaming, boiling—your vegetables/grains/etc. for longer periods of time will soften many foods that are especially hard or coarse. Brown rice can be softened by cooking it in more water for a longer period of time. So instead of cooking 1 cup of brown rice in $2\frac{1}{2}$ cups of water, cook it in 3 cups of water. Let the rice simmer for forty minutes instead of thirty minutes. Short-grain brown rice cooks softer than long-grain brown rice.

When trying to soften vegetables and/or fruits like carrots or apples, it's important not to add too much extra water. Instead, cook them in the same amount of water for a longer period of time by lowering the fire (or heat) and allowing a simmer. This will prevent the essential vitamins and minerals from being leached out. You don't have to sacrifice nutrient density while making your food easier to chew. Purchasing softer varieties of certain produce—such as buying yellow transparent or Macintosh apples instead of Winesap or York Imperial apples—can be helpful. Cutting or chopping food into smaller pieces can also aid in making hard food easier to chew and swallow.

Nuts are nutrient-dense foods that should be included in the diet of all vegetarians. Many types of nuts are excellent sources of iron, calcium, and zinc. However, many seniors are discouraged from consuming them because without strong and healthy teeth, nuts are difficult to eat. One thing my grandmother likes to do is to grind her food in a grinder, which she bought especially for the purpose of making food easier to chew. She uses her grinder most often for nuts—raw almonds, in particular. Then she adds the ground nuts to her cereal and other dishes. This is a perfect technique for making tough or hard foods easier to eat. Nutbutters are another alternative.

DAILY MEAL PATTERN GUIDELINES FOR THE VEGAN SENIOR

Refer to the Daily Meal Pattern Guidelines given in Chapter 4, page 47. Seniors who are cautious of their weight should focus on the lower-range serving numbers. When choosing the specific foods in accordance with these guidelines, refer to the charts in Appendix A. They will help you select the richest sources of calcium, vitamin B_{12}, and vitamin D.

Remember to consume adequate amounts of fluid per day, and a daily multivitamin. Whole grain foods rich in fiber are especially recommended for preventing constipation. Seniors who suffer from conditions such as heart disease, cancer, or others discussed in Chapters 12 through 18 of this book should implement the food guidelines recommended to combat

Table 10.2. Sample Menu		
Breakfast	*Lunch*	*Dinner*
2 pieces homemade biscuits	1 bean patty sandwich on whole wheat bread with lettuce/ tomato	1 cup spaghetti
½ cup scrambled tofu		½ cup "meaty" vegetarian spaghetti sauce
½ cup oatmeal		
1 cup fortified soymilk/ soy beverage	1 cup soy yogurt with 1 oz ground nuts	1 cup collard/mustard/ turnip greens
1 cup strawberry/kiwi/ banana salad	2 medium nectarines	1 large cup tossed salad with ½ cup chickpeas
	1 cup fresh vegetable juice	1 whole wheat dinner roll
		1 cup fruit juice

their conditions. For example, a woman who has a history of colon cancer should be sure to emphasize cruciferous vegetables and soyfoods in her diet. Table 10.2 offers a sample one-day menu for the vegan senior.

TIPS FOR EASIER AND HEALTHIER VEGETARIAN EATING

There are steps that you can take to lighten your burden when it comes to preparing or obtaining balanced meals. The following sections offer helpful suggestions so that you can enjoy healthy cooking and eating.

Preparation of Meals

Preparing meals can become a difficult task for the very aged, as eyesight dims, hands become shaky, and/or certain conditions make it next to impossible to get into the kitchen. Here are some helpful tips for easy meal preparation:

- Purchase a crock pot or a slow cooker. Entire meals can be made easily in this wonderful piece of equipment.

- Use a blender, food processor, or grinder to chop, dice, mix, and knead many foods. A food processor can help with numerous tasks, from making salads to mixing and kneading dough for biscuits and bread.

- Purchase nutritious ready-to-eat foods like whole grain cereals and breads, canned fruits packed in their own juices, and frozen vegetables.

- Cook for more than just one meal and freeze the food in small batches for re-heating at a later date. Foods that can be frozen include some casseroles; vegetable greens (mustard greens, collards); spinach; whole grain muffins; and pancakes.

- Learn several quick and simple, yet nutritionally balanced recipes. Some excellent examples are chili bean tacos and macaroni salad.

- Use the stove timer if you tend to be forgetful or to burn food often.

- Arrange cabinets to make food easily accessible. Have foods placed in a certain order so that you will know where everything is.

- Become familiar with using a microwave, since it can re-heat and cook food at over twice the rate of the oven or stove.

Food Assistance Programs

There are several food assistance programs for seniors who are unable to purchase or prepare their own food. For example, food stamps are provided through state social services or welfare agencies by the U.S. Department of Agriculture. The coupons are used like cash to purchase food and seeds. Seniors, who are eligible, will find that food stamps can greatly increase their purchasing power.

Congregate meal programs (such as those run by local churches, charities, or social centers) are available in many areas. They are located in places where seniors can come to receive free meals and to socialize with others. Transportation to these specific sites can be arranged. There is also a home delivery program known as Meals on Wheels, through which volunteers bring prepared meals to permanently or temporarily home-bound seniors. These programs are open to any person who is sixty or older, regardless of income level. However, priority is given to those who have the greatest financial and social needs.

Vegetarian meals are not readily provided through the above-mentioned assistance programs. You have to specifically ask if a vegetarian meal can be provided. Your local vegetarian society can be of service too, by providing information and working with you to get vegetarian meals.

Residents of nursing and retirement homes can also obtain vegetarian meals; according to the Nursing Home Reform Law, it is a resident's right. In most cases, speaking to your dietitian or food-service supervisor about your vegetarian preferences should be enough to arrange for vegetarian meals. If the meals are unpalatable, the Vegetarian Resource Group, the Vegetarian Nutrition Practice Group of the American Dietetic Association, or the Physicians Committee for Responsible Medicine can provide your institution with nutritional information on and materials for preparing delicious and balanced vegetarian meals. Addresses and phone numbers of these organizations are provided in the Resource Directory of this book, beginning on page 251.

Finally, don't forget that family, friends, and neighbors can serve as some of the best assistance programs. Many older adults do not like to ask for help, as they feel they are a burden on those closest to them. But family and friends often want to help out—that's part of truly loving someone. They can help to purchase and prepare food, and they can provide strong encouragement to eat it.

Many older adults already enjoy very active and healthy lives, and many more can if they learn to change harmful habits and to incorporate a balanced diet into their lifestyle. Vegetarianism is a wonderful way to help maintain optimal health during the golden years. By following vegetarianism, you can help your body prevent chronic diseases such as heart disease, cancer, diabetes, and osteoporosis. Constipation may be relieved by following vegetarianism and/or by eating certain vegan foods. Furthermore, research indicates that risk for arthritis and dementia may even be reduced by consuming a plant-based diet. These health benefits during the senior years certainly prove that the vegan diet enhances life.

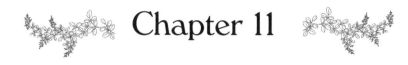

Chapter 11

Eight Essentials for Life

As a child, Natasha Allan hated finishing her spinach and always resisted her 9:30 P.M. bedtime. However, there were some parts of her routine that she liked, such as her nighttime prayers and those evening bike rides with her sister. Natasha was a disciplined and healthy child. Then the college years came. "All-nighters" were common and fast food was convenient. If Natasha decided to spend time outdoors, it was usually to bake herself tan. Cigarettes and alcohol were a favorite weekend combination. Her lifestyle had changed for the worse.

Upon reaching full adulthood, Natasha felt sluggish and stressed. She hated being dependent on unhealthy substances for fun, and found that her body was not as fit as she desired. So Natasha decided to change. After attending a community class on vegetarian nutrition, she became a vegan. In addition, Natasha altered her daily schedule to include more sleep, began a fitness program, and rediscovered her spirituality. Now, as a 40-year-old wife and mother of two, a successful businesswoman, and a vegan for fifteen years, Natasha is once again a healthy woman, known for her vitality and positive outlook.

As children, many of us were not allowed to stay up late into the night. We were punished if caught with a cigarette or alcohol. Eating "yucky" vegetables like spinach and squash was mandatory at dinner. We were taught to say our prayers before bedtime and when we awakened. And we were encouraged to go outside and play.

As adults, we tend to put away all of those childhood ways. We not only stay up late at night, but there are times when we stay up *all* night. We delight in the fact that we can smoke, drink, and eat whatever and whenever we please. Prayers . . . well . . . many of us save those for Thanksgiving, Christmas, Passover, and the other so-called religious holidays. Playing outside has been replaced by the countless times that we walk to and from our cars each day. What we do not realize is that those childhood practices were health-promoting and disease-preventing.

It's time to go back to some of those old routines. This chapter will briefly discuss eight essentials that promote health and wellness. If we take the time to consider these eight essentials for life, we are likely to start adding years to our lives and life to our years.

GOOD NUTRITION

No one can experience optimal health without following a balanced diet. Nutrition influences every aspect of our lives, whether we realize it or not. Our physical and mental well-being are either compromised or enhanced by our nutritional status. Unfortunately, many people do not recognize the numerous health benefits of adopting a vegetarian lifestyle. They don't think about the fact that most meats and meat products are high in fat and cholesterol and contain no fiber.

Many individuals, including the majority of today's health professionals, still do not truly believe that a vegetarian diet is any better than a meat-based diet. Despite the fact that vegetarians have a lower risk and incidence of obesity, high blood pressure, heart disease, cancer, diabetes, osteoporosis, and foodborne illnesses, they are not convinced or impelled to move toward vegetarianism. Furthermore, although a balanced vegan diet is even lower in saturated fat, contains no cholesterol, is high in fiber, and is rich in antioxidants and other beneficial components, veganism is hardly ever recommended. Those of us who do the research realize that veganism makes good sense. It allows nature to help us to grow physically strong, to prevent disease, to promote wellness, and to protect the animal kingdom and our planet.

ADEQUATE REST

All of us know that we should get adequate rest, but it doesn't always happen. Since we cannot pinch time from work or from our daily chores, we steal it from our rest time. We have always been told that seven to eight hours of sleep are necessary in order to be healthy. However, we consider ourselves lucky if we get five or six hours of rest. Of course, not all of us need eight hours of sleep to feel rested; each individual is different. For the most part, the younger you are, the more sleep you need. But most of us will feel and function best with seven to eight hours of sleep.

Sleep disorders are not uncommon. Insomnia is the dreaded "I" word; over 1 million Americans suffer from this frustrating condition. The *Merck Manual of Medical Information (Home Edition)* explains, "Insomnia isn't a disease—it's a symptom that has many causes, including emotional and physical disorders and medication use." For many of us, it all begins when we try desperately to empty our minds of work, bills, marriage tensions, parenting worries, etc. The failed efforts to relax stress us even more. We restlessly turn to look at the clock every couple of minutes. If we're fortunate, we finally fall asleep, only to be awakened in four hours by the annoying sound of the alarm.

You may be lucky enough not to suffer from insomnia. However, like countless others, you may still feel unrested after a full night's sleep. Don't despair, for there are several *drugless* things that we can do to improve our chances of attaining a sound sleep.

First, do not eat a large meal right before bedtime. Large or heavy meals can actually prevent us from feeling rested in the morning, even if we sleep our needed hours. How? Well, the body has to digest the food that it just received, so instead of resting and relaxing, the digestive organs must labor. After such a night, we not only awake feeling unrested, but we do not hunger for a healthy breakfast. Quite differently, something light before going to sleep, such as a piece of fruit or a beverage, will do no harm.

Second, learning how to relax yourself and to relieve stress before you go to bed is very important. Physical exercise, such as a brisk walk outside, followed by a warm shower, is one way that you can help reduce anxiety and prepare your body for a good night's rest. You also should take time to move your mind away from the stressful events of the day and the expectations of tomorrow. Live just one day at a time and leave the troubles of tomorrow for tomorrow. Reading or having someone read to you helps to relax and soothe the mind. A massage by a spouse or other family member will relieve tension. Quiet music, or even nature sounds such as ocean waves, can be soothing. Meditating on positive thoughts or comforting places also encourages relaxation. Some people find that warm liquids before bedtime (decaffeinated, of course) help to induce restful sleep.

Why is adequate rest so important? Clearly, an unrested and sleepy person is an irritated person. Just think back to how many times you told someone, "Look, I did not get a lot of sleep last night, so please. . . . " But more fundamentally, the body gets a chance to rejuvenate and repair itself during sleep. The less sleep you get, the more likely you are to catch whatever illnesses are lurking around work or school. Adequate rest and sleep are actually immune system enhancers. Considering the following list of physical and mental benefits of a healthy amount of sleep, you should alter your schedule to allow for seven to eight hours of sleep per night:

- Repair and maintenance of tissue.

- Removal of wastes that may inhibit normal functioning.

- Feeling alert and energetic while awake, not weary or fatigued.

- Improvement of work efficiency—physical and mental.

- Improvement of concentration abilities.

- Attainment of a healthier attitude; less agitation and irritability.

- Increased prevention of illness.

So despite your busy and hectic schedule, try to set aside time for some overdue sleep, and see if it will improve not only your physical, but your mental, emotional, and social feelings of well-being.

FRESH AIR

When it comes to obtaining fresh air in today's widely polluted world, it feels like there's little we can do. Air has been contaminated to such an extent that aside from being a giver of life, it can be the cause of death. Cities are usually the places where the poorest air quality is found. Despite the grim reality, we must learn to do the best we can with what we have. Every step toward a cleaner air environment counts. This includes avoiding places in which we know the air quality is extremely poor, such as smokers' lounges or recently painted and constructed areas. And, if you are able to make the choice, live as far from the city and as near to nature as you can. Living close to nature includes keeping house plants, which help to provide oxygen.

You and your family may want to consider purchasing an air treatment unit for your home. Be sure to look for a unit that removes particulates, such as dust, mold, and dander, as well as toxic chemical gasses, such as those released from paints, plastics, and pesticides. There are many types of units from which to choose. These air treatment systems are helpful for people with allergies and for sensitive pets, as well.

Smoking is one of the major contributors to air pollution. Every year, millions of Americans die from diseases related to smoking. Lung cancer, heart disease, and respiratory difficulty are just a few. Both the smokers and those around them suffer. Smoking is an addictive and deadly habit, but it can be overcome. If you are a smoker, for the good of your own body and those around you, it is paramount that you find an effective way to quit.

PURE WATER

Water, just like air, is vital to life; without water, nothing can live for very long. Unfortunately, we have a severe problem with water pollution today. In *Everyday Cancer Risks and How to Avoid Them: Effective Ways to Lower Your Odds of Getting Cancer,* author Mary Kerney Levenstein states,

> *Each year in the United States over 70 billion gallons of hazardous waste are generated and 'dumped.' Much of this waste winds up seeping through the soil into both surface and groundwater. More contaminants are added from water pipes that leach lead, vinyl chloride, asbestos, cadmium, copper, and iron in toxic amounts.*

Severe water contamination was experienced firsthand by Milwaukee residents. In 1993, 400,000 people were infected by contaminated water, 4,000 of whom were hospitalized and 100 of whom were fatally sickened. The culprit was a microscopic parasite called *Cryptosporidium.* Contamination with this bacteria occurs when minute amounts of animal feces somehow get into surface waters. Unfortunately, *Cryptosporidium's* unique structure makes it difficult to filter out.

It's not just *Cryptosporidium* that we have to worry about. Tap water can easily contain toxic and cancer-causing chemicals such as lead, arsenic, and pesticides. That leaves us, the American water consumers, with the job of learning how to protect ourselves and our families.

A good way to get cleaner water at the convenience of your tap is to purchase a water filter. But before you run out and buy just any filter, there is some work to do. Different filters serve different purposes; you need to know what kind of contaminants are in your water. If you are on a city or public water line, you can call your water supplier for information on the contaminants. You can also get your tap water tested by your water company or the Environmental Protection Agency (EPA). The EPA is the way to go if your water comes from a private well; the hotline number is (800) 426–4791.

The manufacturer of a filter will usually list on the box the types of purification that the filter offers. Make sure that the filter you select has been certified by the National Sanitation Foundation (NSF) International. Although a water filter won't ensure a 100-percent guarantee that all contaminants will be removed from your water, it certainly will help reduce your risk of becoming ill. You will feel a whole lot better every time you or your family members turn on the faucet to get a glass of water.

Purchasing bottled water might be the first thing that pops into your mind when it comes to avoiding contamination. However, 25 percent of the bottled water that we pay for in the store is just tap water that has simply been filtered for taste. In addition, it is important to keep in mind that filtering water gets rid of some suspended particles, but it does not remedy bacterial problems. It is possible for bacteria to grow within bottled-water containers, if the water has been stored in high-temperature warehouse conditions for a long time.

Water composes over 50 percent of the body. It should be the beverage we drink most abundantly. Generally, it is recommended that the average adult drink six to eight (8-ounce) glasses of water per day. An insufficient fluid intake can lead to dehydration. According to Frances Sizer's and Eleanor Whitney's *Nutrition: Concepts and Controversies,* the symptoms of severe dehydration quickly progress from thirst to weakness, exhaustion, delirium, and, finally, death. Even moderate dehydration makes you more susceptible to colds and to heart problems caused by changes in electrolyte balance. So first we must do our best to obtain pure water, and then we must do our best to drink plenty of it. Photocopy the Fluid Intake Chart on page 255 and stick it on your refrigerator. It will serve as a reminder for you to drink more water and, by placing a check in the appropriate box every time you drink a glass of fluid, you can keep track of how much fluid you are getting.

PROPER SUNLIGHT

Imagine a world with no light, only darkness—an eternal and everlasting night. That doesn't sound too exciting. It probably even sounds depressing, especially for those of us who love to bask in the sun. Fortunately, we do not have to wonder if the sun is going to rise tomorrow. But we should wonder whether we are getting too little or too much sun. Both ends of the spectrum can be dangerous, even fatal.

We are quite aware of the hazards of overexposure to the sun. Health literature is simply bursting with information on how to avoid getting burned, literally and figuratively. For those of us who still feel inclined to bake ourselves in the sun, here's more. Overexposure to the sun can cause heat stroke or heat exhaustion, resulting in fever, chills, weakness, shock, and even death. And sunburn really does age the skin. Wrinkling, elastosis (yellow discoloration with small yellow nodules), and pigment alterations are definite negative consequences. You might not have to go for that facelift if you just take care not to get chronic overexposure to sunlight. Of course, the worst consequence is malignant skin cancers.

Because of the countless occurrences of sunburns, sun poisoning, and skin cancers, you would be lucky to find an article relating the *benefits* of sunshine. As a result, some of us might have forgotten the many benefits of sunshine. But that is also very detrimental to our health. First, sunlight activates the production of vitamin D in our bodies. As vitamin D is not plentiful in foods, the sun is a key source. In addition, the sun is a bactericide and a fungicide, so it helps to prevent infections. The sun also aids in preserving our mental health, as a lack of sunshine can lead to depression. (See "Feeling SAD Without the Sun," below.)

Feeling SAD Without the Sun

Seasonal affective disorder (SAD) is a depressive condition that has been linked to lack of light. It is most common during autumn and winter months. The risk of acquiring this disease is greater in parts of the world where there is very little sunlight—sometimes as little as one hour per day—during the winter season. This occurs at very northern and southern latitudes. But SAD can affect an individual who is house-bound or who stays indoors (away from natural light) for a disproportionate amount of time. SAD is apparently more common among women than men.

Some researchers believe that SAD is a result of improper melatonin secretions. Our pineal gland normally secretes considerable amounts of melatonin—a hormone that aids rest and recovery—during the night. Sunlight inhibits the production of this hormone during the day, which is a good thing because an over-abundance of melatonin can negatively affect mood and normal functioning (concentration, socialization, appetites, etc.). By residing too much in the dark, the body's chemical productions and secretions are thrown off.

SAD proves that our bodies crave light. Among other remedies, people who suffer from SAD can seek *light therapy*, during which they are exposed to full-spectrum fluorescent lighting during the morning and evening. Of course, obtaining natural sunlight in adequate amounts *before* illness occurs is the healthiest route of all.

Most of us have a tendency to think, "If a little is good, then more is better." Usually, too many of those fat-free cookies teaches us otherwise. Overindulgence is rarely a good thing; balance and temperance will do much to preserve life. So a healthy dose of sunlight—not too much and not too little—is vital to our well-being.

FREQUENT EXERCISE

Many of us find that one of the most difficult things to accomplish during the day is exercise. That's unfortunate, as exercise is one of the most won-derful and beneficial things that we can do for ourselves. Some of us tend to shun exercise, always scheduling it into tomorrow's plans. And what are our excuses? "I am just too busy and too tired. By the time I come home from work and do what needs to be done around the house, that's exercise enough for me." That, of course, would be true if we still lived in the *Little House on the Prairie* days, when daily work in and around the home included physical, often back-breaking activities like scrubbing laundry against boards and plowing the field. But it is time for a reality check: we do not get that type of exercise from the chores we typically do. Now, if your routine involves frequently mowing the lawn, pulling weeds, garden-ing, and cleaning out the garage, then you are doing pretty well.

The bottom line for most of us is that we need to move it. Exercise will improve health and help prevent the onset of disease. In fact, it is so impor-tant that I will go as far as to say that a life without motion will eventually lead to a motionless life. If you sit most of the day, join a fitness program or schedule daily walks. Find an indoor track that you can use on cold or rainy days. Aerobics classes are fun, as well as healthy, and are available at many different levels of intensity. These are only a few of many exercise routines from which to choose.

Do not feel that you have to be a specific weight or have a certain amount of strength to start exercising. There is something for everyone. If you need to start slowly because of health restrictions or previous injury, sign up for a beginner's yoga class, in which you learn invigorating stretch-es and positions, and give some time each day to a comfortably-paced walk. Or try water aerobics, which provide a wonderfully stimulating and low-impact exercise environment.

HEALTHY RELATIONSHIPS

Healthy relationships are essential for a happy and healthy life. As John Donne wrote long ago, "No man is an island." No person truly stands alone. The human touch is just as critical to life as water, air, sunshine, and food.

For most of us, the problematic issue is not establishing relationships, but establishing *healthier* relationships, whether between husband and wife, mother and daughter, friend and friend, etc. We need to think about the dynamics of our present relationships, if they help or harm us. An unhealthy relationship leaves a person feeling worthless, hopeless, guilty, and ashamed. Emotional and physical ailments occur. The results are so devastating that they may negatively affect the individual for the rest of her life. The cycle of abuse, guilt, shame, and comfort, followed by more abuse, guilt, and shame, continues to go round and round not only in the life of the abused person, but also down through subsequent generations.

There is a variety of reasons why women remain in unhealthy relationships: financial need; emotional attachment; pure fear of leaving; distorted belief that the abusive relationship is normal. Whatever the reason, understand and realize that if you are being hurt, you are not being loved. Heed these words found in 1 John 4:18, "There is no fear in love; but perfect love casteth out fear; because fear hath torment. He that feareth is not made perfect in love." He that causes you to fear does not love you.

A healthy relationship gives love; it does not take love away. It allows you to grow and expand, educationally and financially. It judges you on your character, not on the shape of your body. When you are sick or frustrated, a healthy relationship nurtures and supports you. Such love wipes away your tears and lifts your burdens. It makes you smile and laugh even when you do not feel too happy.

Holistic health cannot be achieved without establishing warm, supportive, loving relationships. As we nurture and are nurtured, we form an intimate bond with life. We are no longer just living an existence, but we are giving life to others and supporting life within ourselves. If you feel that you're being mistreated, seek help through good friends and/or professional counseling.

A HEALTHY MIND

Indeed, the mind is a powerful instrument, and the relationship that exists between the mind and the body is amazing, to say the least. We get queasy before a test. Our hands sweat and our speech falters when we are introduced to someone special. Some of us lose our appetites when we become depressed, while others eat like food is going out of style. The bottom line is that mental stress physically affects us. Properly managing stress is instrumental in the preservation of our health.

Some researchers conclude that the root of 50 to 95 percent of our physical symptoms are due to our emotions. Put another way, in their book *The*

Health Effects of Attitudes, Emotions, and Relationships, Hafen and coauthors state, "The way we react to what comes along in life can in great measure determine how we will react to the disease-causing organisms that come along. The way we emote—the feelings we have and the way we express them—can either boost our immune system or weaken it." The way we deal with emotions and with illness is the major determinant of outcome.

Stress, particularly negative stress, has severe effects on our health. In *Stress and the Woman's Body,* authors Hager and Hager state, "Stress then not only contributes to the development of various diseases in the body, but also inhibits the ability of the body to fight disease." Research studies have found that stress can cause a rise in blood pressure, induce gastrointestinal distress and disease, and make us more susceptible to infections and other diseases. A 1985 study, done by Peavey, Lawlis, and Goven, looked at the effect of relaxation techniques on the immune response. At first, they found that subjects who were classified into the high stress group had low immunity. But after interventions with biofeedback-assisted relaxation, these same subjects improved their coping skills and their immune responses. Biofeedback involves monitoring certain vital functions, such as heart rate, blood pressure, brain activity, etc. The practitioner then teaches the client certain relaxation practices—for example, meditation, visualization techniques. The client uses these techniques to mentally control the physiological stress reactions, and can watch the monitors and see the reduction in stress effects. This is very self-affirming.

In order to experience optimal health, we must have a positive mindset. The following suggestions will help you on your way to facing what life brings you in a healthy and optimistic manner:

- Do not get upset over trivial things; put things in perspective.

- Always be courteous to others; respect for others will make you feel good about yourself.

- Respond kindly to criticism; use your listening skills.

- Do not talk about others; negative thoughts yield negative feelings.

- Do not go to bed angry; make peace with yourself and others before closing your eyes to sleep.

- Make an effort to think positive, happy thoughts; "mind over matter" can actually work.

- Smile as much as you can; it's a simple way to tell yourself that things are okay.

- Do not get involved with people who undermine you; surround yourself with goodness, wherever possible.

- Mind your own business; stay focused on your path.

- Use relaxation techniques during times of frustration: self-talk; quiet time alone for prayer/meditation; a relaxing walk on a beach or park trail.

- Have a support system; find someone you can trust and with whom you can talk, cry, laugh.

- Regularly engage in physical activity; the exertion releases tension and invigorates the mind and body.

Spirituality also has a wonderful impact on mental and physical health. According to Hafen and coauthors (mentioned previously), "People with a deep sense of spirituality . . . have a purpose, they enjoy a sense of meaning in life, and they have a broader perspective. Spirituality buffers stress; people with a deep sense of spirituality are not defeated by crisis. They are able to relax their minds, elicit the relaxation response, and heal more quickly and completely." Indeed, a relationship with God involving prayer, faith, love, hope, and trust enables us to cope more effectively in the stressful world of today.

Health cannot be obtained without following a lifestyle that includes the eight essentials briefly discussed in this chapter: good nutrition; adequate rest; fresh air; pure water; proper sunlight; frequent exercise; healthy relationships; and a healthy mind. Nourishment comes from many sources, not just off a plate. In combination with each other, the eight essentials offer a *holistic* approach to healthful living.

Part Three

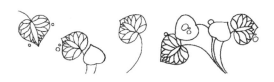

The Vegetarian Advantage Over Chronic Disease

*Education is the best medicine
and prevention is the best cure.*

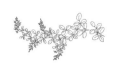 Chapter 12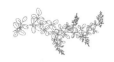

Heart Disease: Caring for Your Cardiovascular System

JoAnna Siegal experienced a heart attack the week after she turned 60 years of age. She survived it, but found herself in shock that it happened to her. We always think such things happen to other people—not ourselves. During her recovery period, JoAnna became quite educated on heart disease, its risk factors, and women's health. She realized just how harmful her family's dietary and lifestyle habits had been.

Before JoAnna's heart attack, the Siegals ate a typical meat-based American diet that was full of saturated fat and promoted high blood cholesterol. Plus, the Siegals had never put much emphasis on exercise, and several family members were smokers. After JoAnna's health problems, the Siegals started making changes. They now follow vegetarianism, exercise regularly, maintain a smoke-free home, and have a new excitement about how they can directly enhance their lives. The Siegals realize that their new lifestyle is not just necessary for long-term health, but also makes life more enjoyable every day.

Cardiovascular disease—including high blood pressure, coronary heart disease (heart attack; angina pectoris, or chest pain), stroke, and rheumatic fever—is not only the number-one killer in America, but it's also the number-one killer of *females* in America. It claimed the lives of some 959,227 people in 1996, more than 505,930 of these being women. In particular, coronary heart disease is the leading cause of death. According to the American Heart Association (AHA), one in five women have some type of heart or blood vessel disease. And the AHA reports that every twenty seconds, someone (male or female) suffers a heart attack; every minute, someone will die from the effects of one. With statistics like these, heart disease is a problem we simply cannot ignore.

The key to reducing the threat of heart disease can be found in *prevention,* and diet plays a large role. It is easy to find, among the advice for a healthier heart, great support for the vegetarian diet. But before we can understand how vegetarianism can improve heart health, we have to understand heart disease itself.

DEFINING HEART DISEASE

Cardiovascular disease refers to all the disorders of the heart and blood vessels that can result in heart attacks and strokes. Atherosclerosis and high blood pressure (hypertension) are two such disorders; they are strongly associated with heart disease. *Atherosclerosis* is the most common form of coronary artery or heart disease. It is characterized by the build-up of plaques along the inner walls of the arteries. Plaque accumulation occurs as a result of repeated fat deposits and damage to the artery walls.

The artery walls are usually very elastic, but as plaque builds up, the blood vessels lose their elasticity. And as the passageways of the blood vessels narrow, blood pressure rises. This increased pressure can cause an artery wall to weaken and balloon out, forming an *aneurysm.* If an aneurysm in a major artery breaks, it causes massive bleeding and, very possibly, death.

When you bleed from injury, your body has a wonderful way of forming clots to stop the bleeding and to aid in cell repair. But unfortunately, plaque can cause your body to form unnecessary clots. The body sometimes responds to the damage occurring in the artery wall by forming clots in the affected area, ultimately making the situation worse. Or a clot can become attached to the plaque in your arteries and continue to grow until it completely shuts off the blood flow to the tissue in that area. A clot can even break off from the site and travel through the bloodstream until it lodges in a vessel that is too narrow to pass through. Picture how the drain in your sink backs up when your bathroom or kitchen pipes becomes clogged. The same thing happens when a vessel becomes blocked.

When a stationary clot has grown large enough to shut off a blood vessel, it is known as a *thrombus.* A coronary thrombus closes off a blood vessel that feeds the heart muscles. A cerebral thrombus closes off a blood vessel that feeds the brain. If a blood clot breaks away from the plaque and starts traveling in the bloodstream, it is called an *embolism.* When the embolism reaches a blood vessel that is too small for it to pass through, it acts like a plug or stopper. If a vessel leading to the heart is stopped up by a clot, a *heart attack* or *myocardial infarction* occurs. And if a vessel leading to the brain is blocked, a *stroke* occurs.

It is obvious that atherosclerosis poses a great threat to health in a number of ways. We must do our best to avoid this process that leads to clogged arteries and, eventually, possible tissue death. Certain factors place us at greater risk for atherosclerosis. They are:

- diabetes*
- diet high in saturated fat*
- heredity (family history)
- high blood cholesterol*
- high blood pressure*

- obesity*
- sedentary lifestyle
- smoking
- stress

Of the nine risk factors listed, five of them—the ones followed by the asterisks (*)—are at least partially related to, if not mostly due to, the food that we choose to eat. This means that we can reduce our potential for heart disease if we carefully monitor our diets. Let's find out how better to do so by delving a little more deeply into issues of weight, blood cholesterol, and "good" and "bad" fats.

LEARNING ABOUT WEIGHT, CHOLESTEROL, AND FAT

Women are three times more likely to suffer from heart disease if they are overweight than if they are lean. Willett and colleagues, in a study published in 1995, reported that the risk of coronary heart disease increases with a rise in body weight. The researchers of this large study found that women who gained weight after the age of 18 had a higher risk for heart disease compared with those who remained lean. The most common causes of obesity are lack of exercise and a diet that contains excessive amounts of fat and calories. Furthermore, it should be noted that android or upper-body obesity is associated with an increased risk of cardiovascular disease.

The Rutger's Guide to Lowering Your Cholesterol by Fisher and Boe discusses the Zutphen study, performed in the 1960s. This study determined a correlation between weight and blood-cholesterol level: a weight increase results in a blood-cholesterol increase, and vice versa. There is also a direct relationship between blood-cholesterol levels and heart disease: as blood cholesterol increases, so does the risk of heart disease.

Blood cholesterol is the means by which fat is transported in the body. When you eat a fatty meal, the liver produces the necessary cholesterol to transport the fat. The more fat and food cholesterol you eat, the more blood cholesterol must be produced to transport it. There is more than one type of blood cholesterol.

LDL-cholesterol (low-density lipoprotein cholesterol) is the carrier that is responsible for taking the fat to the tissues. On the way to the tissues, low-density lipoproteins (LDLs) can lodge in the arteries and accumulate. It is this build-up of fat and cholesterol that forms that harmful plaque. Therefore, LDL-cholesterol is usually referred to as the "bad" cholesterol.

There is another carrier of fat called *HDL-cholesterol* (high-density lipoprotein cholesterol). High-density lipoproteins (HDLs) transport fat away from the tissues so that it can be excreted. HDL-cholesterol is known as the "good" cholesterol.

In general, we should follow a diet that promotes less LDLs and more HDLs. You can easily have your cholesterol levels checked through lab analysis of a simple blood test. Here are some numbers to look for: desirable total cholesterol is under 200 (milligrams per deciliter); desirable LDL-cholesterol is less than 100; and desirable HDL-cholesterol is greater than 45.

Fat and Cholesterol Intakes

Most Americans consume well over the daily recommended levels of fat and cholesterol. This is because meat, eggs, and dairy foods—the major protein sources for Americans—contain lots of fat, especially saturated fat, and cholesterol. The American Heart Association recommends that 30 percent or less of your daily total calorie intake should come from fat. (Optimally, your fat intake should account for between 20 and 25 percent of your caloric intake.) Most Americans consume from 35 to as high as 45 percent of their calories from fat.

Saturated fat is the most solid and the most dangerous type of fat. The AHA recommends that saturated fat intake should be limited to less than 10 percent of your daily calories, while the polyunsaturated and monounsaturated fats should comprise 10 percent each. The average American receives greater than 13 percent of his or her calories from saturated fat, and less than 10 percent from each of the other types of fat. This is not a healthy proportion.

Finally, the AHA suggests that daily cholesterol intake should be 300 milligrams or less. Just one egg contains 213 milligrams of cholesterol, while 1 cup of egg salad contains 629 milligrams of cholesterol. It is not difficult for most Americans who consume eggs, meat, and dairy products to consume too much cholesterol.

The "Good" Fats

Considering all of the dangers that are associated with saturated fat and cholesterol, it is easy to think, "I'd be best off if I simply avoided all fats." That's not true; our bodies need fat. Furthermore, reasonable amounts of unsaturated fats are actually health promoting. Polyunsaturated fats are believed to *decrease* the risk of heart disease by reducing platelet aggregation (or the formation of clots).

In the early 1980s, the relationship between heart attacks and fish oil—a polyunsaturated fat—was studied in the Eskimo population. The Greenland Eskimos have a significantly lower incidence of heart disease than the average Americans or those who consume Westernized diets. Through research, scientists were able to pinpoint that the Eskimos' low incidence of heart disease was due to their greater intake of fish oil, which provides polyunsaturated fats. Fortunately, fish oil is not the only good source of polyunsaturated fatty acids. Most vegetable oils are also excellent sources, including canola, corn, and soybean oils.

Monounsaturated fatty acids also have been found to reduce the incidence of heart disease. Olive oil has become increasingly popular because it is high in monounsaturated fat and contains little saturated fat. Populations who use olive oil as their primary source of fat, such as Mediterranean peoples, have been found to have lower incidences of heart disease. Surprisingly, some of these populations consume more fat than the recommended 30 percent of calories per day, yet still have less cardiovascular disease.

BENEFITTING FROM VEGETARIANISM

Long ago, the research community confirmed that vegetarians have a lower incidence of heart disease than meat-eaters. In fact, some studies report that vegetarians have as much as a 50-percent reduction in the incidence of heart disease. It is important to realize that the vegetarian advantage is well-documented.

Researchers Burr and Butland observed 10,896 British individuals—4,671 vegetarians and 6,225 nonvegetarians—over a period of ten to twelve years. They specifically studied the incidence of heart disease and published the results in 1988, reporting that the vegetarians had significantly lower incidences of death from heart disease. Similarly, the Tromso Heart Study concluded that vegetarian Seventh-day Adventists had lower incidences of heart disease than nonvegetarians did. These are only two of many studies that have come to the same conclusion—vegetarianism promotes better cardiovascular health.

How does vegetarianism—especially veganism—combat heart disease? First, it encourages weight reduction if you are overweight, and the maintenance of a desirable body weight if you are at your proper size. Next, it lowers elevated cholesterol levels, and contains more polyunsaturated and monounsaturated fats (as opposed to saturated fats), as well as high amounts of soluble fiber. Third, vegetarianism emphasizes foods that contain lots of antioxidants. Finally and obviously, vegetarianism completely avoids animal products, which can directly jeopardize our heart health. Let's examine these explanations in more detail.

Weight Issues

Weight loss alone is one of the most effective ways to lower elevated blood-cholesterol levels and to reduce your risk of heart disease. Vegetarianism not only promotes weight loss, but multiple studies have shown that vegetarians tend to weigh less and are closer to their desirable body weights than meat-eaters. One study done by Levin and associates found nonvegetarians to have a 19.5-percent prevalence of obesity, while vegetarians had a 5.4-percent prevalence of obesity. That's a significant difference. Chapter 14 gives important guidelines for losing weight.

Blood-Cholesterol Levels

Lowering your weight is one way to lower your cholesterol. But even if you are not obese, you may have high blood cholesterol. Specific dietary choices make a difference. Researchers West and Hayes conducted a study that investigated the relationship between diet and blood-cholesterol levels in vegetarians and nonvegetarians. The results of the study clearly indicate that the vegetarians consumed less food cholesterol and saturated fat, and thus had lower blood-cholesterol levels than the participants who consumed meat, fish, or fowl once a week or more.

Vegans have even lower blood-cholesterol levels than other vegetarians (lacto-ovo- and lactovegetarians). West and Hayes found that the lacto-ovo-vegetarians had lower cholesterol levels than the meat-eaters, but that the vegans had the lowest cholesterol levels out of all participants. And confirmation of the benefits of veganism has continued to mount.

Resnicow and colleagues published a study in 1991 that strongly supported a vegan diet for individuals with heart disease. The purpose of the study was to compare the differences in diet and lipid levels between vegans and omnivores. Thirty-two vegan Seventh-day Adventists and thirty omnivores agreed to participate in this study. (Fourteen of the subjects were female.) Results showed that the vegans consumed approximately 70-percent less saturated fat than the omnivores, and had lower blood-cholesterol levels. The status of the vegans' health was even more positive than the researchers had expected.

Also, soluble fiber has been proven to be effective in lowering blood-cholesterol levels and, thus, your risk of heart disease. The body is unable to digest fiber, which is a complex carbohydrate. After we eat it, we excrete it. In the process of elimination, fiber binds to fat and cholesterol molecules, and both are then excreted from the body. The different types of soluble fiber are: gums, found in fruits; hemicellulose, found in oats; mucilage, found in barley; and pectin, found in legumes. Fiber is found only in plant foods. Naturally, vegetarians eat more fiber than meat-eaters, since their diets are based on plant foods. Resnicow and associates' research, mentioned previously in this section, concluded that the vegetarian participants consumed 45 grams of fiber per day, while the nonvegetarians consumed only 20 grams of fiber per day. The nonvegetarians in this study served as a good sampling to represent most Americans, who consume approximately 10 to 23 grams of fiber on a daily basis.

The leading health organizations in the United States currently recommend increasing fiber intake by 50 to 100 percent, which would mean ingesting approximately 30 to 35 grams of fiber per day. The table on page 238 in Appendix A identifies foods that are high in soluble fiber and lists the grams of fiber that each food contains. Such foods will contribute to a healthy blood-cholesterol level.

Antioxidants

The vegetarian diet is rich in antioxidants, including beta-carotene, vitamin C, and vitamin E. Antioxidants—or nutrients that work against the harmful process of oxidation in the body—are best known for their role in preventing cancer. Therefore, antioxidant activity is discussed in detail in Chapter 15, which covers issues of cancer and dietary prevention. However, it is important to briefly highlight the role of antioxidants in heart health, as they are instrumental in the prevention of atherosclerosis, as well.

Recently, researchers found that LDL-cholesterol that has been oxidized—combined with oxygen—is more likely to build up in the arteries than cholesterol that has not been oxidized. (The process of oxidation produces free radicals, which are unstable molecules that are destructive to the body.) Antioxidant vitamins not only help prevent LDL-cholesterol from depositing in the arteries, but they also protect LDLs from being oxidized. Some studies looking at the intake of antioxidants and the incidence of heart disease in different populations have concluded that the individuals who consumed the most antioxidants had the lowest incidence of heart disease.

The best food sources of antioxidants are also vegan foods. See Table 12.1 for a list of the top vegan foods that are rich in the particular antioxidants listed. Obviously, the vegetarian diet promotes greater consumption of vegetables, fruits, nuts/seeds, and plant oils—all of which are rich in antioxidants. This seems to be yet another reason why vegetarians have less heart disease than meat-eaters.

Avoidance of the Harmful Effects of Animal Products

Research has clearly linked the consumption of animal protein—meat, eggs, and dairy products—to an increased risk of death from heart disease. A study performed by Snowdon, Phillips, and Fraser reports that both men and women who eat red meat daily have a 60-percent greater chance of dying from heart disease when compared with those who consume red meat less than once a week. The study's results could not be attributed primarily to differences in lifestyle because all of the participants followed the Seventh-day Adventist way of life.

More recent research is showing that meat's effect on heart health might have something to do with iron. Meat is the only source of *heme iron* (for an explanation of heme and non-heme iron, refer to page 55). Research such as that done by Ascherio and colleagues has found an association between the body's heme iron stores and an increased risk of coronary heart disease. *Non-heme iron,* found primarily in plant foods, is better regulated by the body than heme iron, and has not been found to increase the risk of heart disease. Further research must be done before a firm conclusion can be made.

Table 12.1. Antioxidant-Rich Vegan Foods		
Beta-Carotene	**Vitamin C**	**Vitamin E**
Carrots	Papaya	Soybean oil
Winter squash	Orange Juice	Wheat germ oil
Cantaloupe	Cantaloupe	Other plant oils
Sweet Potatoes	Broccoli	Green, leafy vegetables
Spinach	Brussels sprouts	Whole grain foods
Dandelion greens	Green pepper	Nuts
Other dark, leafy vegetables	Grapefruit Juice	Seeds

Another possible reason why meat intake might cause or worsen heart disease is that red meat is a major source of *methionine* in the diet. Methionine, an essential amino acid, breaks down into a compound called *homocysteine.* Elevated levels of homocysteine repeatedly have been found to be associated with an increased risk of heart disease. The Physicians Health Study (all male participants), conducted by Stampfer, Malinow, Willet, and colleagues and published in the *Journal of the American Medical Association* (1992) found that individuals with the highest levels of homocysteine were three times more likely to suffer from heart attacks than those who had the lowest levels of homocysteine. Folic acid, vitamin B_6, vitamin B_{12}, and, most importantly, a low meat intake can help to keep homocysteine at a harmless level.

It's not just meat that promotes heart disease, but dairy and eggs as well. Avoiding all animal products is a healthy move. A study conducted by Toohey and colleagues, published in 1998, looked specifically at African American vegans and lacto-ovovegetarians to determine if the vegans had lower blood pressure and other heart disease risk factors. The results of the study showed that while the vegans and the lacto-ovovegetarians had similar blood pressures, the vegans had a better lipid profile and a significantly higher intake of nutrients that are associated with a lower risk for cardiovascular (heart) disease.

In summary, you can greatly reduce your risk of heart disease by eliminating meat, dairy products, and eggs from your diet. This dietary decision will significantly cut the amounts of saturated fat and cholesterol that you ingest. In *Diet for a New America*, author John Robbins explains that by reducing your meat, dairy, and egg consumption by 10 percent, you reduce your risk of heart attack by 9 percent; by reducing your meat, dairy, and egg consumption by 50 percent, you reduce your risk of heart attack by 45 percent; and by eliminating meat, dairy, and eggs from your diet, you reduce your risk of heart attack by 90 percent.

RECOGNIZING SPECIFIC HEART HEALTHY FOODS

As more and more research is conducted on heart health, vegan foods are being recognized for their benefits. Two particular food types deserve special attention in this chapter. They are nuts and soyfoods.

Nuts

Recently, nuts have gained media attention as studies in prominent medical journals such as the *New England Journal of Medicine* report on their ability to lower blood-cholesterol levels and, thus, to reduce the risk of heart disease. Nuts are not only high in mono- and polyunsaturated fats, but they are also rich in fiber, arginine, vitamin E, and magnesium, all of which have been found to help protect the cardiovascular system.

One of the first studies that suggested nuts' ability to lower the risk of heart disease was conducted by Fraser and colleagues and published under the title, "A Possible Protective Effect of Nut Consumption on Risk of Coronary Heart Disease." In this Adventist Health Study that included 26,473 individuals, consuming nuts five or more times per week was found to provide protection against heart disease. Researchers were surprised, as nuts have always been avoided because of their high fat content. The study showed that the benefits of the mono- and polyunsaturated fats in nuts supersede the disadvantages of consuming their total fat.

Another research project, conducted by Prineas and associates, involved 41,837 women, aged 55 to 69 years. The participants were asked how frequently they consumed a 1-ounce serving of nuts. The researchers found that those who consumed nuts more frequently had a lower incidence of death from heart disease.

Sabate's study published in the *New England Journal of Medicine* attracted a lot of publicity and scrutiny. Participants were placed on one of two diets. Both of the diets met the recommendations of the National Cholesterol Education Program. The only difference between the two diets was that one incorporated walnuts, while the other did not. The researchers were able to conclude from the results of the study that the inclusion of walnuts in the diet has a greater cholesterol-lowering ability than a regular low-fat, low-cholesterol diet without walnuts.

The above described studies clearly indicate that nuts should be a regular part of our diets. Considering all of the different ways that you can incorporate nuts into your diet, and all of the different varieties available, the regular consumption of nuts is not difficult at all. See page 227 for a few ideas.

Soy and Soy Products

When it comes to heart health, soybeans and other soy products are shooting to the top of the list. Research shows that populations who eat soy suffer from fewer heart attacks. On May 12, 1998, the American Heart Association of Northeast Ohio, in conjunction with the Cleveland Dietetic Association and the Ohio Soybean Council, presented an informative seminar entitled "Soy & Cardiovascular Disease Treatment: What We Know, Where We Must Go." Dr. James W. Anderson, a medical doctor and soy researcher, discussed exciting research on several ways that soy can protect against cardiovascular diseases.

Not only does soy lower blood cholesterol, but it has antioxidant properties and it decreases blood clotting. Soy's isoflavones, which are specific plant chemicals, seem to be the responsible components. It is a good idea to consume at least one soyfood rich in isoflavones per day. For a list of several soyfoods and their isoflavone contents, see page 242.

LOOKING AT LIFESTYLE

Is it really the vegetarian diet that is protective against heart disease, or is it the healthy vegetarian lifestyle? After all, vegetarians tend to be health conscious in many areas. Well, we can safely say it's both. A study done by Dean Ornish and colleagues was designed to answer the question, "Can lifestyle changes reverse coronary heart disease?" The researchers found that following a low-fat vegetarian diet, complemented by regular exercise, the cessation of smoking, little or no alcohol, and the performance of relaxation techniques, was characterized by a 24.3-percent reduction in total blood cholesterol, and a 37.4-percent reduction in LDL-cholesterol.

In Ornish's study, the participants who followed the vegetarian diet also experienced a 91-percent decrease in the frequency of *angina pectoris*— pain in the chest associated with heart disease. Quite differently, the omnivorous group experienced a 165-percent increase in the frequency of angina! A regression of coronary artery disease was found in the subjects who adhered to the recommended lifestyle changes and followed the vegetarian diet. As a matter of fact, the better the adherence to the changes, the more regression that was observed.

PREVENTING HEART DISEASE

After reading this chapter, you probably feel an urgency to take good care of your cardiovascular system. In order to do this, I strongly recommend the ten pointers listed below:

• Consider becoming a vegan, if you have not already made this change.

• Eat plenty of antioxidant-rich fruits and vegetables.

• Consume one serving of nuts daily.

• Eat plenty of foods rich in soluble fiber.

• Consume soy and soyfoods, which are rich in isoflavones.

- Maintain a desirable body weight.

- Use fats sparingly. Olive and canola oils rich in mono- and polyunsaturated fats should be used, instead of saturated fats such as margarine, butter, and lard.

- Regularly engage in physical activity.

- Do not smoke.

- Learn to cope with stressful events positively.

Numerous studies have shown the benefits of a vegetarian diet in the prevention and treatment of heart disease. Plant foods are rich in the right components, such as mono- and polyunsaturated fats, soluble fiber, and antioxidants. They are also low in the right components—saturated fat and cholesterol. Do not wait until you are forced to change your life because of cardiovascular illness. Now is the perfect time to get healthy by going vegan.

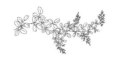

Chapter 13

High Blood Pressure: Learning About the Force of Life

Meegan Langford, a 52-year-old married woman and mother of three teenage boys, had a hectic life but felt rather fine. That's why, at her annual doctor's appointment, she was surprised to learn that she was suffering from hypertension—chronic high blood pressure. In order to reduce her blood pressure, Meegan chose to make several life changes, including becoming a vegan. The vegan lifestyle helped Meegan to lose some extra weight, to cut down on fat intake, and to implement a healthier daily routine. Meegan found herself making time for regular exercise and stopped that light smoking habit she had held onto for years. Her blood pressure returned to a normal range without dependency on pharmaceutical drugs. Deciding to go vegan was the best thing that Meegan Langford did for herself in a long, long time.

High blood pressure is a condition that many Americans do not know they have. It rarely manifests itself in identifiable symptoms. Yet in the United States, more than 50 million people over 6 years of age have high blood pressure. In 1996, hypertension killed 41,634 Americans and contributed to the deaths of about 202,000. Prevention and treatment of this chronic disease is crucial to health, and diet is an important factor. This chapter will discuss how vegetarianism serves as a beneficial lifestyle for healthier blood pressure, but first, let's explore what hypertension is and how it affects the body.

DEFINING HYPERTENSION

Blood pressure is the force of life. It's your blood pressure that is responsible for pushing the blood through your blood vessels so that your tissues can get their supply of nutrients. The pressure that your blood exerts against the walls of the blood vessels must be maintained within a specific range in order to maintain optimal health.

High blood pressure can be explained through a simple metaphor. Imagine holding your garden hose over your precious flower garden, and then shouting to your son or daughter to turn on the water. Instantly, the hose shoots from your hands and slithers uncontrollably like a snake, spouting a damaging stream of water. It plunges into the soil and starts to dig a deep hole. Upset and wet, you quickly attempt to grab hold of the hose while yelling, "Turn it down! Turn it down! It's on too high!" Your child hears your frantic cries and reduces the surge of water. Only then are you able to restore order to your activity and gently water your garden by adjusting the hose to a fine spray.

Just as heavy water pressure can destroy your lovely garden, high blood pressure places too much strain on your arteries, thus damaging them and increasing your risk of obtaining many different diseases. Chronic high blood pressure is called *hypertension.* It is diagnosed by obtaining a blood pressure reading at your health-care professional's office. This reading will yield two numbers: first your systolic pressure, and then your diastolic pressure. Systolic pressure is the amount of pressure placed on the walls of the arteries when the heart muscle contracts, while diastolic pressure refers to the pressure against the walls of the arteries when the heart muscle relaxes. A healthy blood pressure, while you are at rest, is approximately 120/80, but anything below 140/90 is considered within the normal range. A reading above 140/90 is diagnosed as high blood pressure. As diastolic pressure increases, so does the risk of heart attack and stroke.

There are several factors that can contribute to the presence and the worsening of hypertension. These include atherosclerosis, obesity, aging, and inherited factors such as family history and race.

Atherosclerosis (A Cause and a Result)

Atherosclerosis is discussed in detail in Chapter 12, which covers heart disease. Here, suffice it to say that atherosclerosis, which involves the build-up of plaque in the arteries and is the most common form of heart disease, is both a cause and a symptom of high blood pressure. Healthy arteries are capable of expanding and contracting, as the heart contracts and relaxes. When plaque accumulates along the arterial walls, the expansion cannot take place. As a result, blood pressure increases and this extra pressure damages the arteries themselves and causes increased stress on the heart. Then, as Frances Sizer and Eleanor Whitney explain in *Nutrition: Concepts and Controversies,* plaques are more likely to accumulate in areas where arteries are damaged, thus making the process of atherosclerosis a "self-perpetuating" one.

The more plaque in the arteries, the greater the chance that tissues will not get the nutrients they need to survive. This can lead to heart attacks and strokes. In addition, poor blood circulation through the arteries reduces the flow of blood to the kidneys. The kidneys actually have a lot to do with controlling blood pressure. Their job is to filter out wastes from the blood and to excrete these wastes through the production of urine. Normal blood pressure is strong enough to push the blood from the capillaries into the kidneys, where it is purified. If blood pressure is too low at this site, because arterial plaques and damage (or other factors) have reduced the flow of blood, the kidneys secrete hormones that tighten blood vessels and increase the water and salt levels in the body. This heightens blood pressure on the arterial walls even more, and also puts greater stress on the kidneys, causing kidney disease.

Obesity

It is important to understand that obesity increases blood pressure. Excessive amounts of fat cause the heart to work harder in order to supply the tissues with their necessary nutrients. Therefore, it is very important for the hypertensive individual to carefully manage her weight. For a discussion on obesity, see Chapter 14.

Other Factors

There are other, uncontrollable factors involved that can lead to hypertension. The first of these is aging; blood pressure generally increases with age. Second, family history makes a difference. Some people have a genetic predisposition for hypertension. If there is a trend for this disease in your family, you should monitor your blood pressure carefully. Finally, race is a contributing factor. Black people are twice as likely as Caucasians to suffer from hypertension; they develop hypertension earlier in life and with greater severity.

BENEFITTING FROM VEGETARIANISM

Learning how to maintain a healthy blood pressure is not only one of the first things that can be done to *prevent* the onset of heart disease, stroke, and kidney disease, but also one of the first things that can be done to *treat* these disorders. Usually, the traditional treatment prescribed for individuals who suffer from hypertension is a lifetime of medication and careful adherence to a low-salt diet. However, there are additional options. While many health professionals are reluctant to advocate a vegetarian diet because they are not familiar with its benefits, ample research has revealed the effectiveness of a vegetarian lifestyle in lowering blood pressure.

Studies reflecting the lower blood pressure of people who adhere to vegetarian diets date all the way back to the early 1900s. However, it was not until the 1970s that an enormous amount of research on the vegetarian diet and its relationship to blood pressure was performed. The results of these studies indicated that not only do vegetarians have lower blood pressure than meat-eaters, but that a vegetarian diet can effectively and significantly lower the blood pressure in hypertensive individuals.

Since blood pressure increases with age, a study conducted by Melby and colleagues, published in 1993, looked at the blood pressure of meat-eaters and vegetarians over 55 years of age. Both Black and Caucasian participants were studied. The vegetarian participants were members of the Seventh-day Adventist Church. The results showed that both the Black and Caucasian vegetarians had lower blood pressures than their omnivorous counterparts. The researchers also found that the longer an individual followed the vegetarian diet, the lower his or her blood pressure was. Thus, they concluded that adherence to a vegetarian diet early in life provides significant dietary protection against heart disease in later life.

Most clinical research looking at the vegetarian diet and blood pressure has studied lacto-ovovegetarian Seventh-day Adventists. However, a study performed to assess the role of a vegan diet on blood pressure was performed by Lindahl and colleagues in Sweden. All of the twenty-nine participants had been diagnosed by physicians as having high blood pressure and were on hypertensive medications. As instructed by the study, the participants followed a vegan diet for one year, during which time they were encouraged to discontinue their use of medication. After the year, twenty of the participants were completely off their hypertensive medications and six were taking lower doses (most commonly, half of their original doses). On the whole, the blood pressures did not decrease dramatically after the year, but it should be noted that the vegan diet was able to replace the use of medications for an impressive number of the participants.

LOOKING AT LIFESTYLE

Despite the evidence supporting the vegetarian diet's role in preventing and treating high blood pressure, most researchers deny that it is the avoidance of meat that is responsible for lower blood pressure. Instead, they attribute the healthier blood pressure to other possible factors, such as lower body weight, reduced intake of salt, and the high potassium level of a balanced vegetarian diet. Furthermore, lifestyle characteristics—for example, regular exercise and abstaining from alcohol—that are common among vegetarians are given all the credit for the generally lower blood pressures. So a 1982 study by Rouse and colleagues researched whether it was solely a vegetarian diet or a general healthy lifestyle that was responsible for the lower blood pressures in vegetarians. They compared two religious groups who observed the same lifestyle but differed in their diets. The results of the study indicated that the vegetarian Seventh-day Adventists had significantly lower blood pressures than the omnivorous Mormons. The conclusion was that lower blood pressure is directly linked to following vegetarianism.

The same researchers decided to do a follow-up study to determine if the vegetarian diet would reduce the blood pressure of healthy meat-eating subjects. This 1983 study published in *The Lancet* reported that after fourteen weeks, there was a significant fall in the blood pressure of the participants who followed the vegetarian diet. The researchers strongly felt that the reductions in blood pressure were completely diet-related. These studies, in conjunction with several others, confirm the therapeutic role that a vegetarian diet plays in the treatment of hypertension.

But is it solely what vegetarians eat that gives them the edge when it comes to blood pressure management? Evidence tells us that both the vegetarian diet and the typical vegetarian lifestyle promote better health when it comes to hypertension and the diseases it causes. The observance of several health-promoting practices enables vegetarians to maintain a desirable blood pressure. For example, the people who choose vegetarianism because of their strong concern for physical health also tend to exercise often, to avoid smoking and alcohol, and to carefully manage their weight. Furthermore, vegetarians do tend to have a higher potassium intake (which is beneficial to blood pressure regulation), while consuming less saturated fat. This simply means that optimal health can be experienced only when you implement a *holistic* change in your way of life, meaning that you attend to all the parts that make up the whole.

PREVENTING HYPERTENSION

There are several ways that we can help our bodies to prevent hypertension. I suggest the following pointers:

- Follow a vegan eating pattern.

- Include plenty of fresh fruits and vegetables in your diet.

- Avoid foods that are high in saturated fat.

- Limit your intake of salt and salty foods.

- Exercise regularly.

- Do not smoke.

- Avoid all beverages that contain alcohol.

- Maintain a healthy weight.

- Train yourself to deal with stressful events in a constructive manner. Stress alone can increase blood pressure to dangerously high levels.

A healthy blood pressure is essential for a healthy life. It is important for you to know what your resting blood pressure is and what it should be. If you have not done so recently, have your blood pressure checked by your health-care professional. A healthy blood pressure is associated with long life expectancy and low risk of heart disease. Situations of illness due to low blood pressure are rare, while hypertension is dangerous. Importantly, don't panic if your blood pressure is over 140/90. Feel confident that there is much you can do to make a positive difference in your health, including following a vegan diet.

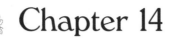
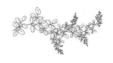

Chapter 14

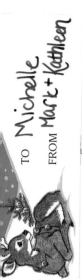

TO Michelle
FROM Mart + Kathleen

besity: Weighing the Weight Issue

Danielle Johnson was in the seventh grade when she saw a picture of herself and decided to make major changes to her lifestyle: "I was huge, weighing in at 191 pounds, and I was only 13 years old." Unhappy with her condition, Danielle started getting serious about losing weight. She began exercising every morning and evening for about an hour, and she made the complete transition to veganism. Danielle explains, "I avoided high-calorie, high-fat foods like sweets, milk, and dairy products, and I cut my portions in half." It took two years, but Danielle lost 70 pounds. She confidently states, "Veganism made a wonderful difference in my life."

I t's hard not to notice that America is getting bigger. No, I'm not talking about more people; I'm talking about more weight on people. There is an upward trend in the prevalence of overweight and obese people in the United States, and that is nothing to brag about. From 1960 to 1994, the number of obese adults jumped from 13 percent to 22.5 percent of the general population. Furthermore, most of this increase has occurred in the 1990s, according to the National Institutes of Health (NIH).

It is now estimated that over 97 million American adults are considered either overweight or obese. That is 55 percent of the population who is placing themselves at risk for health problems. The good news is there is something we can do about it. Obesity is preventable and, for most individuals, weight loss can be successfully achieved without drugs or surgery. Making permanent changes in lifestyle and eating habits can bring the majority of individuals to a healthy body weight.

Many females will admit that they weigh more than they would like to. Most have legitimate concerns, while some are just too influenced by unhealthy trends of "skinniness" in our culture. It seems to come naturally to females to worry about their weight. This is probably due to many factors, including society's preoccupation with the female body. While a woman's weight is of vital importance for her health and well-being, I would also like to emphasize that inner beauty should always be considered of utmost value. When approaching the issue of weight loss, it should be addressed from the angle of improving health, rather than from fitting into society's often warped definition of what every woman should look like. If you are concerned with obesity, it is important to learn about proper weight assessment, so that you can make healthy decisions about your body.

ASSESSING YOUR WEIGHT

The National Institutes of Health have provided guidelines for assessing weight. There are three key measures to consider: body mass index (BMI); waist circumference; and risk factors for diseases and conditions associated with obesity.

Body Mass Index (BMI)

The BMI figures determine the appropriateness of a person's weight. This scale gages weight according to height. You can determine your BMI by using Table 14.1; the data was organized by the National Institutes of Health and the National Heart, Lung and Blood Institute, and has been printed in Dr. David Heber's *The Resolution Diet.* Simply find your height in the far left column and continue along the line until you find your weight. Then trace straight up to the top row of the table for your BMI number.

According to NIH, a BMI of 19 to 25 is considered healthy; a BMI of 25 to 29.9 is considered overweight; and a BMI of 30 or more is considered obese. NIH recommends that an individual with a BMI over 30 should lose weight. Individuals with BMIs between 25 and 30 may not need to lose weight if they do not have other risk factors, but should carefully avoid any further weight gain. It is important to note that muscular individuals may have BMIs greater than 25 without health risk.

Waist Circumference

The circumference of your waist is another important measurement that should be considered alongside your BMI. NIH reports that people who have BMIs between 25 and 34.9 and waist circumferences greater than 40 inches in men and 35 inches in women increase their health risks. An inappropriate waist circumference (common in apple-shaped individuals) alone can increase your risk of disease. NIH states, "People whose weight is concentrated around their abdomens may be at greater risk of heart disease, diabetes, or cancer than people of the same weight who are pear-shaped." So not only do you have to consider how much you weigh, but also where the fat is located.

Conditions Associated with Obesity

The final key to weight assessment is the presence or risk of certain diseases and disorders associated with obesity. If you already have any of these conditions or a propensity for them, you have to be extra careful to maintain a healthy body weight. The excessive fat that defines obesity can lead to numerous health complications. The following is a list of the health hazards associated with being obese:

- adult-onset (type II) diabetes

- arthritis

- depression

- gynecological irregularities

- heart attacks

- high blood-cholesterol concentration

- high blood-triglyceride concentration

- hypertension (including pregnancy-induced hypertension)

- increased number of physical injuries

- increased risk for cancers of the breast, uterus, ovaries, gallbladder, bile ducts, and cervix

- low self-esteem, feelings of worthlessness

- respiratory problems

- strokes

- varicose veins

You may be surprised at the cancer information provided in the previous list. In the report *Understanding Adult Obesity,* published in November of 1993, NIH explains that when compared with women who maintain healthy body weights, obese women are more likely to die from gallbladder, breast, uterine, cervical, and ovarian cancers. This is a frightening realization that many of us don't want to hear. But by learning about these risks, we can be further motivated to do something about excess weight.

IDENTIFYING THE CAUSES OF OBESITY

Is it nature or nurture? Genetics or eating habits? What is responsible for obesity? This debate most likely will continue as long as time lasts. However, we can find some reasonable answers when we take *both* nature and nurture into consideration.

An individual can definitely inherit a tendency toward excessive weight gain. This can be related to slow metabolism, glandular problems, or other

Table 14.1. Body Mass Index

BMI	19	20	21	22	23	24	25	26	27	28	29	30	31	32	33	34	35	36
Height								Weight in Pounds										
4'10"	91	96	100	105	110	115	119	124	129	134	138	143	148	153	158	162	167	172
4'11"	94	99	104	109	114	119	124	128	133	138	143	148	153	158	163	168	173	178
5'0"	97	102	107	112	117	122	127	132	138	143	148	153	158	163	168	174	179	184
5'1"	100	106	111	116	122	127	132	138	143	148	153	158	164	169	174	180	185	190
5'2"	104	109	115	120	126	131	136	142	147	153	158	163	169	175	180	186	191	196
5'3"	107	113	118	124	130	135	141	146	152	158	164	164	169	175	180	186	191	203
5'4"	110	116	122	128	134	140	145	151	157	163	169	175	180	186	192	197	204	209
5'5"	114	120	126	132	138	144	150	156	162	168	174	180	186	192	198	204	210	216
5'6"	116	124	130	136	142	148	155	161	167	173	179	186	192	198	204	210	216	223
5'7"	121	127	134	140	147	153	159	166	172	178	185	191	198	204	211	217	223	230
5'8"	125	132	139	145	152	158	165	172	178	185	191	197	203	210	216	223	230	236
5'9"	128	135	142	149	155	162	169	176	182	189	196	203	209	216	223	230	236	243
5'10"	132	140	147	154	161	168	175	182	189	196	202	209	216	222	229	236	243	250
5'11"	136	143	150	157	164	171	179	186	193	200	208	215	222	229	236	243	250	257
6'0"	140	147	155	162	170	177	185	192	199	207	214	221	228	235	242	250	258	265
6'1"	144	151	158	166	174	181	189	196	204	211	219	227	235	242	250	257	265	272
6'2"	148	155	164	171	179	187	195	203	210	218	225	233	241	249	256	264	272	280
6'3"	152	160	168	176	184	192	200	207	216	224	232	240	248	256	264	272	279	287
6'4"	156	164	172	181	189	197	205	214	222	230	238	246	254	263	271	279	287	295

Clinical guidelines on the identification, evaluation and treatment of overweight and obesity in adults. National Institutes of Health; National Heart, Lung and Blood Institute (1998).

physiological aspects of the body. And then we learn a lot of our habits through parental modeling. For example, a woman who struggles with overeating told me how her dad would go into the grocery store for two things and end up with three or four bags of groceries. He would spend hours shopping for food. The woman soon realized that she, too, would stay in the store for long periods of time, picking out food after food. She was unconsciously mimicking his behavior. Modeling behavior—learning from example—is something that all humans do. Parents who eat unhealthily are more than likely to raise children who follow the same eating patterns.

And yet, it is not just the genetics and the influence of family members that has a direct affect on our weight. The media, with its constant advertisement of high-fat, high-calorie foods, certainly plays a role. The availability of fast food—most of which is laden with fat—is no help either. Many Americans decide to frequent fast food restaurants rather than cook a decent, balanced meal.

Table 14.1. Body Mass Index

BMI	37	38	39	40	41	42	43	44	45	46	47	48	49	50	51	52	53	54
Height								Weight in Pounds										
4'10"	177	181	186	191	196	201	205	210	215	220	224	229	234	239	244	248	253	258
4'11"	183	188	193	198	203	208	212	217	222	227	232	237	242	247	252	257	262	267
5'0"	189	194	199	204	209	215	220	225	230	235	240	245	250	255	261	266	271	276
5'1"	195	201	206	211	217	222	227	232	238	243	248	254	259	264	269	275	280	285
5'2"	202	207	213	218	224	229	235	240	246	251	256	262	267	273	278	284	289	295
5'3"	208	214	220	225	231	237	242	248	254	259	265	270	278	282	287	293	299	304
5'4"	215	221	227	232	238	244	250	256	262	267	273	279	285	291	296	302	308	314
5'5"	222	228	234	240	246	252	258	264	270	276	282	288	294	300	306	312	318	324
5'6"	229	235	241	247	253	260	266	272	278	284	291	297	303	309	315	322	328	334
5'7"	236	242	249	255	261	268	274	280	287	293	299	306	312	319	325	331	338	334
5'8"	243	249	256	262	269	276	282	289	295	302	308	315	322	328	335	341	348	354
5'9"	250	257	263	270	277	284	291	297	304	311	318	324	331	338	345	351	358	365
5'10"	257	264	271	278	285	292	299	306	313	320	327	334	341	348	355	362	369	376
5'11"	265	272	279	286	293	301	308	315	322	329	338	343	351	358	365	372	379	386
6'0"	272	279	287	294	302	309	316	324	331	338	346	353	361	368	375	383	390	397
6'1"	280	288	295	302	310	318	325	333	340	348	355	363	371	378	386	393	401	408
6'2"	287	295	303	311	319	326	334	342	350	358	365	373	381	389	396	404	412	420
6'3"	295	303	311	319	327	335	343	351	359	367	375	383	391	399	407	415	423	431
6'4"	304	312	320	328	336	344	353	361	369	377	385	394	402	410	418	426	435	443

Consider, too, that many social events are centered on food. We celebrate the arrival of a new employee with food. We celebrate the departure of an old employee with food. We have a Christmas party at a restaurant, a big Christmas dinner at home, and we go to a few treat-filled Christmas parties on the side. All of these events contain lots and lots of food.

The stresses of life may cause us to turn to food as a comforter. Ice cream, cookies, cakes, and pies somehow seem to have a natural ability to calm our nerves and perhaps relieve our frustrations. Many of us have not been taught good survival techniques, so instead of dealing with frustrations in a positive manner, we may turn to food, drugs, alcohol, depression, or hundreds of other things in an attempt to cope. Overindulging will take its toll on well-being.

Whether you believe that you fall more heavily on the nature or the nurture side, or whether you think it's an equal combination of both, one thing is for sure: People who are obese tend to consume more calories than they burn up. Most of those calories come in the form of very processed and refined foods that contain high amounts of calories and fat, while offering few nutrients. Potato chips, soda-pop, candy, and desserts are just a few of the foods that fit into this category.

In addition to consuming too many calories, most obese people do not regularly engage in physical activity. Modern technology and culture has made it simple for us to accomplish many things without exerting much effort. Ultimately, for many of us, daily labor usually involves more sitting than anything else. We just never find the time to go for a walk, take a jog, or use the bicycles that are collecting dust in the garage. Eventually, the guilt about the lack of physical activity lessens, and we become comfortable with our inactivity. That doesn't change the fact that exercise is crucial for the maintenance of a healthy body and optimal weight.

In our rushed culture, we also tend to consume a lot of food in a little time. Label-reading is inconvenient, and many of us skip meals and have irregular eating times. Consuming high-calorie, high-fat foods, including meat, dairy foods, eggs, and products made with these items, makes the challenge to our bodies even worse. And let's face it: We don't tend to condition ourselves to say "No thank you, I'm not hungry," when we're not hungry. So, before we are able to catch our breaths, we find that we have put on more pounds than we would have liked. Knowing the risk factors and identifying them within our own lives can help either to prevent ourselves from becoming obese, or to target the habits we need to break in order to lose weight.

BENEFITTING FROM VEGETARIANISM

Vegetarianism has found its way into the lives of many women who desire to reduce their weight. Numerous studies have found that the majority of vegetarian women are closer to their ideal body weights than are their meat-eating counterparts. For example, a study by Janelle and Barr, published in 1995, reported that vegetarian participants weighed less and had significantly lower BMI values than meat-eating participants. In addition, the estimated percentage of body fat was lower in the vegetarians.

In addition, you may recall a study discussed in Chapter 12, performed by Levin and his fellow researchers. The study concluded that the prevalence of obesity was 5.4 percent among the vegetarian participants, and 19.5 percent in the meat-eating participants. And a 1978 study by Sanders and Associates, publised in the *American Journal of Clinical Nutrition*, found vegans to be lighter in weight and to have smaller amounts of body fat than omnivores of the same height.

A vegetarian diet is typically lower in fat and higher in fiber than the standard American meat-based diet; animal products are high in saturated fat and cholesterol, and they have no fiber. A *vegan* diet is most effective when it comes to achieving or maintaining healthy weight.

TAKING THE FIRST STEPS TOWARD WEIGHT LOSS

Despite the fact that the odds of being obese are greater for meat-eaters, many of us vegetarians and vegans can testify that we, too, are guilty of engaging in harmful eating practices, and we might even weigh a little more than we would like. I am not talking about eating potato chips at a picnic or enjoying a piece of pie once in a while. I am talking about the chronic over-consumption of high-calorie, high-fat, and low-nutrient vegetarian foods.

There are numerous "bring-on-the-bulge" products in which a vegetarian can indulge. Does the following case scenario ring a couple of familiar bells? You are late for work and you surely do not have much time for preparing a healthy breakfast. So you grab a quick bowl of frosted cereal, telling yourself, "The sugar will give me energy for the hectic morning I'm about to face." When lunch rolls around and you have thirty minutes, *McDonald's* French fries and apple pie fit right into your time constraints, along with two of *Taco Bell's* bean burritos—just for balance. You wash that down with a tall soda-pop. When you get home a little late that evening, you decide not to cook a big dinner; the *Top Ramen* noodles in the cupboard and the *Tator Tots* in the freezer will do just fine. Dessert is *Tofutti* and a few cookies.

All of the foods just mentioned can be considered vegetarian, and some are actualy vegan, but they should not be a regular part of the diet. Foods that contain lots of calories and fat but little vitamins, minerals, and other nutrients, should be eaten infrequently. They can and will help to make you much larger than you desire to be. Low-fat eating is emphasized in the majority of weight-loss plans because fat contributes the greatest number of calories per gram. One gram of fat contains nine calories, whereas one gram of protein or carbohydrate has four calories.

Once you have identified what your optimal weight is, it is time to learn how you can achieve that weight. People have attempted and continue to attempt to lose weight in numerous ways. There are the magic pills; special oils; delicious milk shakes; "eat next-to-nothing" diets; "eat whatever you want" diets; and the "Doctor, please cut it off, staple it shut, or wire it closed" solution. The products and processes are endless! In certain circumstances, they are dangerous. In truth, there is no quick fix. So learning to lose the weight means accepting that a healthy, slow process that involves a commitment to self-control and exercise is the most effective route.

Positive Mental Attitude

Before you ate that ice cream or devoured too many potato chips, you probably heard a little voice inside trying to convince you that you really should not be splurging. That little voice probably was followed by another little voice that was trying to convince you that you deserved to splurge since you had such a hard day. Maybe you told yourself that this would be the last time you would eat junk-food, or maybe you made a silent comparison between yourself and Mrs. So-and-So and thought, "I'm not that bad." When I counsel clients on weight loss, I tell them that success begins in the mind. Proverbs 23:7 tells us, "As a man thinketh in his heart so is he." And so, the first step in learning to lose weight is to learn to control your thoughts and to develop a positive mental attitude. Here are five tips for maintaining a healthy, optimistic approach to your weight loss program:

- Read, see, and listen to as much encouraging information about weight loss as possible. For example, read books like *Thin for Life* by Anne Fletcher and Jane Brody (Chapters Publishing, Ltd., 1995), and join support groups such as community groups and Overeaters Anonymous, so that you can hear success stories and benefit from group pep-talks.

- Maintain a positive view of yourself that exists outside of how much you weigh. You can do this by keeping actively social with friends who make you feel invigorated and confident, and by continuing hobbies or avocations at which you are good, such as music lessons, painting, or working with children.

- Know the thought patterns that trigger harmful eating practices. For example, you may find yourself thinking, "A few potato chips aren't going to make a difference in the long run." When you feel yourself challenged, strengthen your determination with motivational self-talk: "If I eat this bag of chips, I will not feel better, I will feel worse about myself. This is the wrong way to deal with my problem."

- Develop a strong support system, which includes positive and loving relationships with family and friends, as well as a healthy spiritual life. Learn to communicate your feelings within this support system. Instead of grabbing a package of cookies after a bad day at work, talk to your spouse, call a friend, or take some time to pray/meditate.

- Never, ever give up. Never tell yourself that you cannot reach your goal, even when you falter. Pessimism *can* be overcome.

Your motivation to lose weight should grow from the desire to make your life a more comfortable and enriching experience. If you consume wholesome, pure foods that do not damage the body or your conscience, you will be a much happier and peaceful person.

Reasonable Goals

If you are serious about losing weight, you must establish your goals. Long-term success is dependent upon short-term commitments. So with each step you take toward successful weight loss, you need to have both long-term and short-term goals. Few of us can tackle a mountain without first succeeding on the hills.

The first goal that you must set is the amount of weight that you want to lose. If you doubt your ability to set an appropriate weight goal, you should seek the advice of a health professional, preferably a dietitian. If you decide to work with a weight counselor, be honest and open about what you desire.

The next goal you need to establish is the period of time in which you want to lose the weight. Again, short-term and long-term goals must be determined. In order to set an appropriate time period for yourself, consider the two basic principles of losing weight: You must eat fewer calories and you must exercise more. In order to lose just 1 pound of fat, you have to eat 3,500 calories less or burn 3,500 calories more. It sounds simple enough, yet it can be very difficult to accomplish.

As a general rule of thumb, expect to lose 1 to 3 pounds a week. This is a healthy rate at which to lose weight. If you are a busy person with less time for physical activity, or if you are unable to engage in physical activity, allow yourself a longer time period for weight loss. Every person has her unique needs and lifestyle. Thus, you should factor in as many variables as you can think of that will affect the time in which you can accomplish your goal.

A Plan of Action

Now that you know how much weight you need to lose and in how much time you desire to lose it, the next step is to determine exactly *how* you plan to lose the weight. In developing a plan of action, you must identify what it is that causes you to overeat or that inhibits you from making healthy changes in your life. So before you start making any changes in your diet or lifestyle habits, keep a diary of your activities and feelings every day for one to two weeks. Write down all of your activities and feelings. For example, you may note, "Felt frustrated because kids and husband left the house a total mess; snacked on six peanut butter cookies while watching TV." From the time you get up to the time you go to bed, it is important that you write down the times that you do certain things: "Snacking on potato chips at 2 P.M.," or "Watching TV from 5 to 8 P.M." Make sure that you log everything you eat, the time of each meal and snack, and the amounts you eat.

The purpose of the diary is for you to get a better idea of what you are doing with your time and why you are doing it. Many of us do not realize that we have extra pockets of time available for us to engage in activities. We might be astonished at how much time we actually waste on unhealthy habits, as well as how intimately our feelings affect our actions. You will begin to identify patterns.

After you have kept a diary for one to two weeks, make a list of the things that you believe you need to change about your lifestyle—eating habits, work habits, physical activity routines, negative thought patterns. The list may include such goals as: gradually eliminating meat products; gradually cutting out milk and dairy foods; avoiding junk foods such as potato chips and donuts; avoiding fried foods; cooking three nights per week; exercising five times per week, in forty-minute intervals; cutting portion sizes; and increasing your intake of fruits, vegetables, and other high-fiber foods.

Next, separate the list into short-term and long-term goals and place them into your desired time frame. Maintain the practice of keeping a diary until you reach your long-term goal. It helps you to track your successes and failures. Thus, three months from the time you start changing your habits, you might be surprised at just how far you have come. Some people choose to write every day, while others find weekly entries more suitable, and still others prefer making notes every two weeks. Just be sure that you write frequently enough to be able to record specific changes in your habits and patterns.

EATING TO LOSE WEIGHT

Most of us agree that a healthy weight-loss program should emphasize more fruits and vegetables and less starchy and/or fatty foods. As far as calories are concerned, vegetables contain the least amount of calories per serving. Consider Table 14.2, which lists vegetarian foods and a breakdown of the major components for each.

If you follow an eating pattern that includes large amounts of fruits, vegetables, and legumes, and less starches and nuts, you are better able to lose weight while still eating healthy. You will find this pattern of eating will allow you to feel satisfied after every meal, as high-fiber foods give

Table 14.2. Vegetarian Food Exchange				
Food	Calories	Protein (g)	Carbohydrate (g)	Fat (g)
Starch/bread (1 slice; ½ cup)	80	3.0	15	1
Legumes (½ cup)	105	7.0	20	trace
Tofu/soy product (½ cup)	150	12.0	12	6
Fruit (1 medium piece; ½ cup)	60	—	15	—
Vegetables (½ cup)	25	2.0	5	—
Nuts/seeds (1 oz)	165	5.5	2	15
Fat, such as canola or olive oil (1 tsp)	45	—	—	5

you a feeling a fullness while providing a healthy intake of essential nutrients. It will establish a foundation for a lifetime of healthy eating.

The guide in Table 14.3 is designed for the vegan female who wishes to lose weight. It tells you how many servings of each food group you should eat per day, for a 1,200-, 1,500-, and 1,800-calorie diet. All of these calorie levels should promote weight loss in most women. If you plan to consume eggs and dairy, you will need to adjust the pattern. For optimal weight management though, I suggest a vegan diet.

Even though weight loss programs put the emphasis on reducing fat intake, remember that it makes no difference what the food sources are when it comes to excessive calories—eventually, excessive body fat will result. Cutting down on fat should not be accompanied by filling up on low-fat foods that still provide excessive amounts of calories.

If you think you will never get used to eating that baked potato without all the cheese and butter, think again. Usually, with time, our taste buds change and we are better able to adapt and enjoy healthier foods. I speak from personal experience. When I first moved in with my grandmother, I

Table 14.3. Vegan Food Pattern for Weight Loss in Women

Food Group	Serving Size	Suggested Number of Servings		
		1,200-cal. Diet	1,500-cal. Diet	1,800-cal. Diet
Whole grain products (bread; cereal; pasta; rice)	1 slice, ½ bagel; ½ cup	4	4	5
Fruits; fruit juices	1 medium; ½ cup chopped; ¼ cup dried; 6 oz	4	4	5
Vegetables (including dark green); vegetable juices	½ cup cooked; 1 cup raw; 4 oz	3	5	5
Tofu; tempeh; low-fat meat analogs	4 oz	2	3	3
Legumes/beans	½ cup	1	2	2
Nuts and seeds (including nutbutters)	1 oz; 2 tbsp	1	1	1
Vitamins B_{12} and D-fortified foods	As specified for food group.	1	1	1

had to get used to eating low-salt cooking. My grandmother has high blood pressure and does not consume much salt. At first, I was constantly struggling against my tendency to grab the salt shaker. Two years later, I wasn't adding salt to my food at all, and truly enjoyed my meals. As a matter of fact, now when I eat meals prepared by people who are not salt-conscious, the food tastes too salty.

CONSIDERING A FEW MORE TIPS

The following sections offer a few more suggestions when it comes to tackling the difficult task of losing weight. First, exercise is key to burning those extra calories. And then, making weight loss a group effort may encourage you to stick to your plan.

Regular Exercise

Exercise is a major factor when it comes to health and fitness. Establishing a regular exercise program is essential when implementing a good weight-loss program, and knowing the type of exercise that you should focus on is important. Aerobic exercise, such as walking, jogging, swimming, and bicycling, performed for at least forty minutes, burns the most fat. Anaerobic exercise strengthens, tones, and develops the muscles; it does not burn fat.

There are many practical and easy ways to increase your physical activity. For example, park in the most distant parking spaces at shopping centers, and whenever possible, take stairs and walk up escalators, instead of taking elevators. Walk to nearby places, instead of driving. If you have trouble finding long spans of time to do exercise, it might be easier to exercise for fifteen minutes in the morning (before work), and then fifteen minutes in the evening. Even a fifteen minute walk during lunch break might be possible.

Strength in Numbers

Working together as a family or a group of friends will encourage your success at losing weight. Most of the changes that you have to make in your eating pattern should also be implemented into the family eating pattern. Too much fat and sugar is not good for anyone, whether they are overweight or not. And exercise is not just for those who want to lose weight, it is for everyone.

So get together with your family or a group of friends and talk about changes that all of you can make to improve your health. Family members and friends should also be your strongest support system and cheering team. Tell them what they can do to help you to keep your commitments and your spirits up.

If you do not have any personal friends or family members to work with you, involve yourself in walking clubs, dancing or karate classes, healthy cooking or low-fat eating classes, or community programs on health or weight loss.

Learn to let go of the "diet" notion. Many people believe that in order to lose weight, a temporary diet must be implemented. And when we think of diet, we usually think of depriving ourselves for a greater good. We think about *eating less,* when we should be thinking about *eating better.* I strongly believe that permanent weight loss is not associated with temporary abstinence, but with healthy and balanced lifestyle habits. The vegetarian—especially the vegan—diet promotes the healthy intake of nutrients without excessive saturated fat and cholesterol. And a holistic approach to nourishment is most effective—it involves more than the food you put into your mouth; it means developing a lifestyle that invigorates and enhances the body, mind, and spirit.

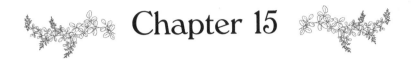

Chapter 15

Cancer:
Practicing Prevention

Charlene Santos panicked when she felt a lump in her breast. Though just 22 years old and a healthy eater—a vegan—Charlene thought, beyond a shadow of a doubt, that she had breast cancer. Charlene immediately made an appointment to see her gynecologist. She explained to her doctor that her mom had a history of polycystic breasts and, while the lump may simply be a cyst, she wanted confirmation. After reviewing several options, Charlene decided to have the lump aspirated by a surgeon and tested for malignancy.

The lab tests came back negative, and Charlene had peace of mind. This terrifying experience, however, made her even more health conscious. She now incorporates more soyfoods, fruits, and vegetables into her daily diet, as these vegan foods help prevent cancer. Charlene is also careful to keep up with her self-exams and her annual doctor's appointments. Prevention and early detection are critically important.

Every year, over 184,000 American women get breast cancer and some 43,000 women die from this terrible disease. In 1996, 257,635 women died from various cancers; of these, 61,731 died from lung cancer alone. Such a frighteningly large number merits the alarmed response that most females experience when the word *cancer* is mentioned. Though cancer is not the number one killer of women, it is the most feared killer of women. And well it should be dreaded, as it takes second place in diseases that claim the lives of females.

Despite the widespread anxiety concerning all types of cancer, many women do not take the necessary measures to decrease their risk of developing them. Cancer treatments improve with each new year, and research is constantly probing for a cure, but *prevention* should be the ultimate goal. This chapter will provide you with the basic facts on cancer and what you can do to prevent it, including following a vegetarian diet.

DEFINING CANCER

What is cancer? Most people would find this question very easy to answer: Cancer is a terrible disease that gradually takes the life of too many of our friends and relatives. Scientifically, though, cancer is a disease that causes the uncontrolled growth of abnormal cells. The textbook definition of cancer is: "A disease in which cells multiply out of control, forming masses (tumors) that disrupt the normal functioning of one or more organs."

Cancer is believed to be initiated by either a physical or chemical event in which an individual is exposed to a particular *carcinogen*—a cancer-causing substance. The carcinogen gains access and takes over cells. It commands the now abnormal cells to make more and more copies of themselves, resulting in the formation of a tumor. Therefore, a *tumor* is an unchecked growth of tissue that has no function. Tumors can be either benign or malignant. A benign tumor usually is not life threatening, while a malignant tumor is very life threatening.

Terminal cancer is most often associated with *metastasis,* which occurs when cancer cells move from the primary site to other sites in the body. Often, the cancer travels via the bloodstream and/or the lymphatic system. Once a cancer has metastasized, prognosis worsens.

There are different types of cancer, each with a specific name to identify the tissue that it attacks. For example, a sarcoma is a cancer that affects muscle, bone, or connective tissue. Leukemia is a cancer that affects the blood cells. Some types of cancer are associated with the female's anatomical and reproductive system. These include cancers of the breast, ovary, uterus, cervix and cervical dysplasia, vagina, vulva, and fallopian tubes.

Breast, lung, and colon cancer are the top three cancers from which women die each year. Though a cure for cancer has not yet been found, treatments are improving. Moreover, there is much that we can do to decrease our risk of obtaining this dreaded disease.

Despite the fact that some of us might be more genetically prone to cancer than others, lots of research is confirming that the way we choose to live and what we choose to eat have dramatic effects on our cancer risk. According to the U.S. Department of Health and Human Services, 80 percent of all cancer is related to lifestyle and dietary habits. Arthur Upton, MD, the former director of the National Cancer Institute, believes that up to

50 percent of all forms of cancer are linked to diet. Many other research studies have found that diet plays a role in 30 to 70 percent of cancers. This news should be enthusiastically welcomed by all, as it allows us to take an active part in preserving our health. The dietary and lifestyle habits that have been shown to be associated with a higher risk of cancer are:

- smoking and tobacco use
- excessive alcohol consumption
- excessive sun exposure
- exposure to environmental contaminants
- little or no fruit and vegetable intake
- high animal (saturated) fat and cholesterol intake
- little or no dietary fiber intake

BENEFITTING FROM VEGETARIANISM

Simply put, people who choose to eat plant-based diets have lower incidences of cancer than those who choose to eat meat-based diets. A study conducted by researcher Frentzel-Beyme and colleagues, published in 1994, found that a vegetarian lifestyle is associated with a substantial reduction in the incidence of *all* cancers, and that the longer you are a vegetarian, the lower your risk of getting cancer is. Researchers concluded that participants in the study who had been vegetarian for twenty years or more decreased their risk of dying from cancer by 50 percent.

Rosy Daniel, the Medical Director of Bristol Cancer Help Centre, summarized a study done by researcher Daniel published in 1994. It involved 11,000 adults. The study reported that vegetarians were 40 percent less likely to die from cancer.

For years, Seventh-day Adventist vegetarians have been recognized for their lower incidence of cancer. As a matter of fact, according to Whitney and coauthors in *Understanding Normal and Clinical Nutrition* (third edition), Adventists have one-half to two-thirds the mortality rate from cancer than the rest of the population, even with the exclusion of cancers linked to smoking and alcohol. Studies looking at the cause of this significant difference have found the Seventh-day Adventists' avoidance of meat and their higher intakes of fruits, vegetables, and grains to be the responsible factors.

It is alarming that more is not done to educate the public regarding this issue. However, things are looking up for the American public as a few health organizations have started publishing the well-established truth about plant-based diets and cancer risks. The American Institute for Cancer Research's "Diet and Health Recommendations for Cancer Prevention"

(1998) includes information that strongly supports a vegetarian diet. The first recommendation is "choose predominantly plant-based diets rich in a variety of vegetables and fruits, legumes and minimally processed starchy staple foods." The report goes on to confirm that a cancer-prevention diet is based primarily on plant foods, as "Strong and consistent scientific evidence shows that vegetables and fruits protect against many different types of cancers." It further discusses how plant-based diets reduce risk of obesity, which is a risk factor for several cancers. These recommendations also advise: the consumption of five or more daily servings of various fruits and vegetables; the consumption of more than seven daily servings of grains, legumes, plantains, roots, and tubers; limited amounts of refined sugar; and "if eaten at all," limited intake of red meat because large amounts of animal products, especially red meats, are linked to cancer.

There are several specific reasons why the vegetarian (especially the vegan) diet is so powerful when it comes to preventing cancer. First, many fruits, vegetables, grains, and legumes contain antioxidants, which battle cancer-causing molecules. Also, beans and other plant seeds contain isoflavones, which serve as antioxidants and play other roles in cancer prevention. In addition, the vegan diet is naturally high in fiber and low in saturated fat. And vegan foods have been found to enhance immunity, while meat and other animal products add unhealthy elements to your diet.

Antioxidants in Fruits and Vegetables

More than likely, you have already heard of free radicals and antioxidants. If so, you are probably aware that free radicals help to cause cancer and antioxidants help to fight it. The process of how free radicals are made and how they work can be quite complicated. (See "Are We Captive to Free Radicals?" on page 169.) We can simplify the explanation by saying that a free radical is an unstable molecule that attacks and damages cells in the body. The production of free radicals is associated with an increase in the risk of cancer. Continuous free-radical attacks can turn a normal cell into a cancerous one. It takes only a single cancerous cell to start the dreadful cancer process, because that cell has the ability to multiply at an enormous and uncontrollable rate. In addition, the cancer cell surrounds itself with a protective covering that the body's immune system cannot penetrate.

Remember, though, that this process started with an unstable molecule. It is at this early stage that antioxidants become important. *Antioxidants* are defined as chemicals that work to change the harmful and unstable free radicals into harmless and stable molecules. Beta-carotene, vitamin C, and vitamin E are antioxidants and are found almost exclusively in plant foods.

Fruits and vegetables are rich sources of beta-carotene and vitamin C, while whole grains are rich in vitamin E.

Vitamin A and the carotenoids are also potent antioxidants. The major food sources for vitamin A include liver, fish liver oil, fortified milk, and eggs. But the vegetarian needn't worry about obtaining enough vitamin A from foods because carotenoids can be converted to vitamin A by the liver. Many plant foods that are rich in color—particularly green, yellow, orange, and red vegetables—are rich in carotenoids and therefore have vitamin-A activity. There are hundreds of carotenoids, but among the best known are beta-carotene, lutein, lycopene, and alpha-carotene.

Several research studies have found that individuals with the highest intakes of carotenoid-rich fruits and vegetables have the lowest risk for

Are We Captive to Free Radicals?

According to *Dynamic Nutrition for Maximum Performance* by Daniel Gastelu and Dr. Fred Hatfield, oxygen molecules within our bodies break down for a number of reasons: as a result of radiation from the sun; in response to ozone, carcinogens, and other pollutants; and even as a result of natural body processes like metabolism and exercise. When an oxygen molecule is altered and loses an electron, it becomes highly reactive and capable of bonding with another molecule, thus becoming a free radical. In its mission to replace the lost electron, the free radical pairs with another and becomes more reactive, beginning a spiral of cell destruction.

Free radicals can harm cell membranes, damage genetic material, and work against healthy immunity. They can alter fats, proteins, and carbohydrates. Research has found that, when uncontrolled, free radicals promote the development of many degenerative diseases, including cancer and heart disease, not to mention the aging process.

We can protect our cells from extensive free-radical damage by increasing our antioxidant intake. Antioxidants neutralize free radicals before they can do much damage. A number of nutrients serve as antioxidants, including vitamins A, C, and E, beta-carotene, selenium, manganese, and zinc, among other substances. Antioxidants are stronger when taken in combination, rather than when taken alone. This is a good reason to take antioxidant supplements.

many cancers, including lung, colon, stomach, esophagus, and oral cancers. Most studies on vitamin A and cancer actually use the carotenoid beta-carotene from fruits and vegetables as the source of vitamin A, or they use vitamin A or beta-carotene supplements. In fact, in an article entitled "Biological Functions of Dietary Carotenoids," author Adrianne Bendich states, "carotenoids have antioxidant potentials which are well above that seen with vitamin A."

The antioxidant power of fruits and vegetables cannot be emphasized enough. The Centers of Disease Control report that individuals who consume five or more servings of fruits and vegetables per day decrease their risk for lung, colon, stomach, esophagus, and oral cancers, when compared with individuals who eat less fruits and vegetables. A study performed by Trichopoulou and associates, published in 1995, found that women who ate more vegetables had a 48-percent reduction in their breast cancer risk, while those who ate more fruits had a 32-percent reduction, when compared with subjects who had lower intakes of these healthful food groups. Another study, performed by LaVecchia and colleagues, looked specifically at the intakes of fruits and vegetables and the incidence of stomach cancer. The researchers concluded that a low intake of fruits and vegetables is associated with a seven times increase in the risk of getting stomach cancer.

There are certain families of fruits and vegetables to which you should pay special attention in order to prevent cancer. Most fruits and vegetables contain vitamin C and beta-carotene, but some are outstanding sources of these vitamins. Citrus fruits, such as lemons, limes, oranges, tangerines, and grapefruits, are extra-rich in vitamin C. Yellow-orange fruits, such as apricots, cantaloupes, papayas, peaches, and pineapples, as well as cherries, berries, plums, prunes, strawberries, and watermelons, are extra-rich in vitamin C *and* beta-carotene.

Dark green, leafy vegetables contain high amounts of beta-carotene. These include such foods as spinach, broccoli, Swiss chard, kale, romaine lettuce, endive, chicory, escarole, watercress, and the greens of collards, beets, turnips, dandelions, and the mustard plant. Yellow-orange vegetables, such as carrots, sweet potatoes, pumpkins, and winter squash, are also great sources of beta-carotene.

Cruciferous vegetables are another food found to be effective in the prevention of cancer. Vegetables from this family contain compounds, scientifically known as indoles, dithiolthiones, and others, that protect your body from cancer. The cruciferous family of vegetables includes: bok choy; broccoli; Brussels sprouts; cabbage; cauliflower; collard greens; kale;

kohlrabi; mustard greens; rutabagas; turnips; and turnip greens. For a list of the top cancer-prevention foods, see the inset below.

Isoflavones in Legumes and Other Plant Seeds

Legumes, especially soybeans, contain high levels of *isoflavones*—a family of plant chemicals. *Genistein* is the primary isoflavone in these foods and, in particular, has been found to decrease the growth of breast and prostate cancer cells. According to *An Alternative Medicine Definitive Guide to Cancer,* written by W. John Diamond, MD, W. Lee Cowden, MD, and Burton Goldberg, genistein inhibits estrogen's ability to promote tumor growth, blocks the functions of some cells that are thought to be responsible for initiating cancer, and may even stop new blood vessels from forming, thus hindering the growth of certain tumors. Genistein is a powerful antioxidant.

Cancer-Prevention Foods

All of the cancer-prevention foods advertised by the National Cancer Institute on its poster boards are vegan foods. Practically every food group in the vegan diet contributes immensely to the prevention of disease, especially cancer. Below are listed the foods that the National Cancer Institute finds to be *highly protective* against cancer:

• cabbage	• cilantro	• licorice root
• carrots	• garlic	• parsnips
• celery	• ginger	• soy beans

And foods that are *modestly protective* against cancer are:

• basil	• cucumber	• thyme
• berries	• flax	• tomatoes
• brown rice	• oats	• tumeric
• cantaloupe	• onions	• whole wheat
• citrus fruits	• oregano	
• cruciferous vegetables	• peppers	

Diadzein is another isoflavone that is found in soybeans and other legumes. Like genistein, diadzein serves to arrest estrogen action, therefore reducing the growth rate of tumors that are dependent on hormones. For a list of isoflavone-rich foods and their approximate isoflavone contents, see Appendix A, page 242.

Fiber in Plant Foods

Fiber is recognized as having a protective effect against cancer. Too little fiber in the diet automatically places you at risk for many medical problems, cancer (especially colon cancer) included. Fiber is very instrumental in helping wastes to be moved quickly through the intestinal tract, thus allowing potential harmful substances that we consume through our foods to be passed out of our bodies quickly. Giovannucci and colleagues found there to be a 50-percent reduction in the risk of colon cancer in individuals who consumed a high-fiber (30 grams daily) diet, as opposed to those who consumed a low-fiber (12 grams daily) diet. And a high-fiber diet is not only instrumental in preventing colon cancer; researcher Gorbach concluded that a low-fat and high-fiber diet reduced the incidence of breast cancer by 16 to 24 percent in his research participants. Fiber also helps to keep the intestinal muscles strong. For a complete summary of fiber's health benefits, see the inset on page 173.

Vegetarians naturally eat more fiber than the average Americans do. Fruits, vegetables, legumes, and grains are the key sources of fiber and the foundations of vegetarian diets. And statistics show that the incidence of both colon and breast cancers are significantly lower in vegetarians than in meat-eaters.

Low Saturated Fat and Low Cholesterol in the Vegetarian Diet

Fat intake—primarily saturated fat, found largely in animal products—has been shown to be associated with increasing the risk of specific cancers such as breast and colon cancers. For example, researchers have found that the amount of fat consumed by a woman seems to be related to her risk of getting breast cancer. This association is explained further by Table 15.1, which identifies the breast-cancer risk per 100,000 women in different countries, and compares it with the average amount of fat that is eaten in their diets. You will note that Thailand and Japan have the lowest incidence of breast cancer, as well as the lowest fat consumption. The breast cancer death rate in the United States is significantly higher, as is the average fat consumption of 146 grams per day.

While there is reliable evidence that fat plays a role in the development of breast cancer, it is important to note that not all types of fat seem to fit into this category. The consumption of olive oil (a monounsaturated fat) instead of other fats has been associated with as much as a 50-percent *reduction* in the incidence of breast cancer. On the other hand, the fat found in meat (saturated fat), particularly red meat, increases the risk of cancer. A six-year study, conducted by Toniolo and colleagues, studied over 14,000 women and found that those who ate $2\frac{1}{2}$ ounces or more of red meats—beef, luncheon meats, lamb, veal, and pork—every day increased their risk of breast cancer by 50 percent. For more on the subject of animal products and cancer, see page 175.

Both the American Cancer Society and the National Cancer Institute recommend that total fat should be limited to less than 30 percent of the total daily calories. Some research studies have shown that consuming 20 to 25 percent total fat is actually more beneficial. This recommendation is important not only because an excessive fat intake is associated with a higher cancer risk, but also because an excessive fat intake will lead to obesity; obesity, itself, is another risk factor for cancer. Just by avoiding too

---

The Benefits of a High-Fiber Vegan Diet

A vegan diet that is high in fiber can positively affect your health in many ways. Such a diet can:

- increase protection against cancer at most sites in the body, particularly cancers that affect the body's membranes and the respiratory and digestive tracts

- lower blood-cholesterol levels

- maintain normal bowel function, regularity; reduce constipation

- prevent diverticulosis of the colon

- reduce blood pressure in hypertensive individuals

- reduce risk of diabetes; improve blood-sugar control

- reduce risk of obesity; assist with weight loss and weight maintenance

Every person should make an effort to consume a considerable amount of fiber daily. The recommended daily minimum is 25 grams.

much fat in your diet, you are likely to reduce your cancer risk from two different directions.

Food cholesterol is another problem. It is a precursor to almost all of the substances known to cause colon and rectal cancer. The relationship between food cholesterol and these types of cancer has been well established. Eggs are a very rich source of cholesterol and saturated fat, as is most meat. Researchers Phillips and Snowdon found that the frequent consumption of eggs was associated with fatal colon cancer; those who consumed eggs five or more days a week had a higher risk of fatal colon cancer than those who consumed eggs less than two days a week. Keep in mind that the vegan diet is the answer to avoiding the repercussions of food cholesterol—plant foods contain absolutely no cholesterol.

Table 15.1. Comparison of Fat Intake With Death Rates From Breast Cancer		
Country	**Deaths Due to Breast Cancer (per 100,000 women)**	**Daily Fat Intake (in grams)**
Australia	18.5	129
Austria	16.0	118
Bulgaria	8.5	65
Canada	23.0	140
Ceylon	3.0	44
El Salvador	2.2	40
Germany	16.5	137
Hungary	13.6	97
Japan	4.0	38
Netherlands	26.0	155
Panama	7.0	57
Poland	11.0	85
Portugal	13.0	66
Switzerland	22.0	137
Taiwan	4.6	42
Thailand	2.0	21
United States	21.0	146

Enhanced Immunity From the Vegetarian Diet

There seems to be increasing proof in medical literature that the functioning of the immune system has a lot to do with cancer prevention. According to McGinn and Haylock, in their book entitled *Women's Cancers,* our immune systems definitely play a large role in determining cancer risk. For example, AIDS (acquired immune deficiency syndrome) is a disease that attacks the body's immune system, and McGinn and Haylock explain that almost 70 percent of individuals with AIDS develop cancer.

If the evidence continues to build in this direction, enhancing the body's immune system definitely will be a central area of cancer prevention. Diet has dramatic effects on the strength of a body's immunity; deficiency in certain nutrients actually suppresses immunity. Among these nutrients are: individual amino acids; folate; iron; pantothenic acid; vitamins A, B_6, B_{12}, and E; and zinc. A proper vegan diet is the best way to get these nutrients through foods.

Avoidance of the Harmful Effects of Animal Products

Even with the large amount of evidence supporting a vegetarian diet in the prevention of cancer, most health professionals tend to believe that the issue lies more with the high intake of fruits, vegetables, and other plant-based foods, rather than in the avoidance of meat. It may indeed be true that the top reasons why vegetarians have lower cancer risks are related to the fact that they are less likely to be obese and that they consume higher intakes of cruciferous vegetables, citrus fruits, and fiber. However, it should not be forgotten that meat, eggs, and milk still contribute to cancer risk; they contain the highest concentrations of known carcinogens. Furthermore, as discussed in the previous material on fat and food cholesterol, meat and eggs contain significant amounts of saturated fat and cholesterol.

In the *International Journal of Health Services,* Samuel S. Epstein explains that due to lack of competent regulation at the federal level, the meat industry uses numerous additives when preparing animal feed. These include antibiotics, pesticides, artificial flavors, and even tranquilizers, industrial wastes, and growth hormones! Surely, the animal products that humans consume are, in turn, contaminated with such substances.

Meat, milk, and eggs contain the highest concentrations of organochemicals that have been linked to promoting cancer. The more animal products we eat, the higher the concentration of these chemicals become in our own systems. Epstein also states, "Even a dime-sized piece of meat contains billions of trillions of molecules of these carcinogens." Naturally, those who eat these products are placing themselves at higher cancer risk.

Roy Hertz, former Director of Endocrinology at the National Cancer Institute and a world authority on hormonal cancer, has expressed much concern about the cancer risk of estrogen-containing feed additives. He believes that no dietary levels of these uncontrolled and unregulated estrogen additives should be regarded as safe. While fruits and vegetables also may be contaminated with certain organochemicals, they do not contain even half of the amount that meat does, and many of the chemicals are lost in the washing and peeling of the produce.

PREVENTING CANCER

Here are the top ways that you can lower your risk of suffering from cancer. They are *daily* suggestions.

- Eat plenty of fresh fruits that are rich in antioxidants such as beta-carotene and vitamin C. Citrus fruits are very high in these nutrients.

- Eat plenty of vegetables, especially cruciferous and carotene-rich vegetables.

- Eat plenty of whole grain products and legumes.

- Drink plenty of water and fruit/vegetable juices.

- Increase your fiber intake.

- Avoid meat and meat products.

- Avoid milk, eggs, and products that include these items in their ingredients.

- Avoid foods that are high in fat, especially saturated fat and cholesterol. Your total fat intake should amount to less than 30 percent of your total calories. (Preferably, 20 to 25 percent of your calories should be from fat.)

- Avoid alcohol and caffeinated beverages.

- Wash all fresh produce well before eating; discard the outer layers of leafy vegetables.

- Maintain a healthy body weight.

If you follow these guidelines, you will be taking an active role in preventing cancer in your body. In this day and age, we cannot afford to be passive about carcinogens in our diets. Women must realize the power they have in affecting their own health.

Cancer is one of the most feared diseases, despite the fact that the medical and health communities are making strides in cancer research. The fact remains that the best cure for cancer is prevention. The vegetarian diet—especially the vegan diet—offers many benefits in fighting off cancer. Such a diet provides high intakes of antioxidants, isoflavones, and fiber; it is low in saturated fat and cholesterol; it enhances immunity. Furthermore, plant-based foods contain considerably less toxic contamination than animal products. So it makes solid sense to become a healthy vegan.

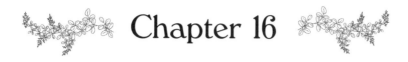

Chapter 16

Osteoporosis: Battling Bone Loss

Felisha Porter, a 29-year-old single female, became concerned about her bone health after her mother's hip fractured. When her mom was discharged from the hospital, she brought home several pamphlets on osteoporosis and its prevention. Felisha took the time to read all of the information her mom had been given, and determined within herself that she would prevent this disease from ever affecting her. The main problem, though, was that all of the prevention material emphasized increasing calcium intake by consuming more milk and dairy products. Felisha had been practicing veganism for over five years and had no desire to change her diet.

Fortunately, Felisha decided to attend a class on vegetarianism that was being offered in her community. At the seminar, she discovered that a balanced vegan diet would not compromise her bone health—it would actually help her to preserve it! There are many vegan foods that can supply adequate calcium intake. In fact, research shows that vegans may require less calcium, as they are likely to absorb it better. Furthermore, vegans have fewer bone breaks and fractures. So Felisha didn't have to change her dietary practices at all.

Osteoporosis is becoming increasingly recognized as a serious disease from which older adults in industrialized nations suffer. In the United States alone, 13 to 25 million Americans have osteoporosis, and one out of five American women over 65 years of age has had one or more bone fractures. The best way for women to increase their bone health is to make healthy dietary decisions, such as following vegetarianism, and to commit to weight-bearing exercises. This chapter will define osteoporosis and explore prevention in detail.

DEFINING OSTEOPOROSIS

Though we do not often consider it as such, bone is a living tissue that is constantly being broken down, rebuilt, and reformed. Bone formation is necessary for normal growth to occur, and for the repair of bone fractures and breaks. There are three basic phases of bone development throughout the life cycle, and these phases overlap. The first phase spans from birth to the early-20s. This time is characterized by rapid growth and development in the length, the width, and the shape of the bones. During the second phase, which occurs between the ages of 12 and 40, the bones become thicker and denser. The final phase begins between the ages of 30 and 40, and continues throughout the rest of life. At this stage, the breakdown of bone takes place at a faster rate than bone formation and, thus, bone loss occurs.

Osteoporosis involves this loss of bone mass, resulting in increasingly porous and fragile bones. Many adult and older persons are afflicted with osteoporosis. The bones are more likely to fracture and break, and they heal at a reduced rate. This disease afflicts women in particular, especially after menopause. The effects of osteoporosis are debilitating, disfiguring, and painful.

The most recognized sign of osteoporosis is an abnormal curvature of the spine, leading to a stooped posture called a *dowager's hump*. This is a symptom of advanced osteoporosis, when 30 to 40 percent of bone mass has been lost. In such a situation, the vertebrae have weakened and deteriorated to the point of collapse. Effects on the spinal column also cause decreases in height; some people lose as much as 5 to 8 inches. But even if an individual's osteoporosis does not manifest itself in this severe way, it is still a significant danger. The most frequent and injurious result of osteoporosis is stress fractures.

In the United States, 80 percent of 14 million hip fractures are due to pre-existing osteoporosis. Twenty percent of these cases result in death within three months. Older people who recover from hip fractures often suffer long-term and extensive physical, emotional, and financial repercussions. It is estimated that our nation spends $1.5 to $2 billion per year on hospitalization, nursing-home care, and outpatient services for victims of hip fractures. National medical cost could be reduced by 20 percent if the incidence of hip fractures decreased.

Diagnosis

According to the *Merck Manual of Medical Information,* osteoporosis can be diagnosed in a number of ways. Often, it is obvious through a physical examination and/or x-rays of the bones that are done when a fracture is present. You can also check the condition of your bones *before* a fracture occurs. This is accomplished most accurately through a dual-energy x-ray absorptiometry (DXA) test; this test will measure your bone density through low doses of radiation (less than those emitted during a common x-ray). The quick exam takes from five to fifteen minutes to perform. Usually, it is reserved for those females believed to be at high-risk for osteoporosis, those whose diagnosis is questionable, and those who require a very accurate assessment of bone density because treatment decisions would be critical.

Specifics on Women's Bone Health

As we age, the rate of calcium absorption decreases and we have to pull reserves from the bones, therefore weakening them. For example, according to researcher Spencer, a woman who is 21 years of age absorbs about 44 percent of the calcium she ingests, while a woman of 51 years may absorb as little as 22 percent of her daily calcium intake.

All people will experience some bone loss due to the aging process. However, women lose bone mass at a faster rate than men. According to Dr. Susan M. Lark, an authority in the field of women's health care and preventive medicine and author of the book *The Estrogen Decision,* during the first five to ten years after menopause, women can lose as much as 1 to 3 percent of their bone mass per year. This is due to the drop in estrogen levels that occur with menopause. Men, on the other hand, have denser bones—they have approximately 30 percent more bone mass than women—and their testosterone enables them to preserve bone mass and strength.

By the age of 60, women can lose up to 40 percent of their bone mass, placing them in a very dangerous condition. Those who have smaller bone structures feel the effects of bone loss more than women who have larger bone structures. Caucasian women, particularly those of Northern European ancestry (such as the Dutch, German, and English), who are 35 years of age or older have a high risk of developing osteoporosis due to their smaller skeletal mass at maturity. Darker-skinned or Black females usually come to maturity at a larger skeletal mass.

The increased loss of bone mass in women is due to several factors. A profound factor is hormonal changes that occur with menopause or a hysterectomy (the surgical removal of the uterus). A loss of estrogen quickens the loss of calcium in the body. Some women make the decision to go on estrogen replacement therapy to restore estrogen levels in the body. But this has pros and cons; see "Considering Estrogen Replacement Therapy" on page 184. In addition, genetics play a major role in determining the rate of bone loss. The top three genetic factors include race, gender, and peak bone mass.

As with other frightening diseases, when it comes to osteoporosis, the best avenue to take is prevention. To reduce your risk of osteoporosis, health professionals recommend that you ingest sufficient amounts of calcium (1,000 to 1,300 milligrams per day). Maintaining a good calcium balance throughout life is essential for optimal bone health. You should also perform weight-bearing exercises—for example, walking, going up stairs, lifting weights—which build bone mass. And, as mentioned previously, some older women take estrogen as a preventive measure, as this hormone naturally protects women's bones.

For those who already have the disorder, taking supplemental calcium and vitamin D seems to aid in increasing bone density. Estrogen and/or pharmaceutical drugs that increase bone mass may be suggested for more severe cases. Physical therapy is helpful to many individuals, as are supportive braces and pain medications. Finally, exercise is strongly recommended to strengthen the muscles (especially the back muscles), which help support and hold the bone structure.

BENEFITTING FROM VEGETARIANISM

As mentioned above, one of the top recommendations for the prevention and treatment of osteoporosis is to provide your body with a considerable amount of calcium. For decades, adequate calcium intake through the consumption of milk and dairy products has been strongly encouraged in the United States as the primary way to prevent osteoporosis. Every year, billions of dollars are poured into the advertising of dairy items as foods that promote bone health.

Yet most health professionals fail to consider why osteoporosis is so prevalent in the industrialized nations where meat and dairy consumption are highest, while it is hardly seen in nations where milk consumption and calcium intake are significantly lower. For example, some African cultures maintain diets that do not include any dairy products and that provide only 175 to 475 milligrams of calcium each day. Still, the people in these cultures have a lower rate of osteoporosis than Americans. Furthermore, according to a study done by Abelow and colleagues that involved participants from several different nations, as calcium intake increased, the number of hip fractures also increased. (The rate of hip fractures helps to determine the prevalence of osteoporosis.)

Many bone researchers have concluded that calcium intake is only one factor in the prevention of osteoporosis, and most likely a minor factor at that. For example, researchers Wachman and Bernstein theorized that the prevention of osteoporosis might have more to do with a plant-based diet versus an animal-protein diet, rather than with copious amounts of calcium-rich foods. There are many ways to decrease your risk of osteoporosis. Yes, an adequate calcium intake is one, but so is an adequate intake of vitamin D, phosphorus, and several other nutrients. Surprisingly, researchers are finding that high protein (generally meat-based) diets can harm our bone health, while soy protein diets can help it.

Could it be that the majority of health professionals and the advertisement world are focusing on the wrong foods for the prevention of osteoporosis and the maintenance of optimal bone health? Dietitians and other health professionals still find it difficult to believe that a vegan diet that excludes milk and other dairy products could support the healthy development of bone, and many have concluded that following such a diet may eventually result in poor bone health and osteoporosis. The vegan diet has been devalued as an inadequate source of calcium; vegans are generally considered at an increased risk of bone disease. But research is strongly showing otherwise.

Negative Effects of High-Protein, Meat-Based Diets

Some researchers have found that bone health may be compromised not as a result of a low calcium intake, but as a result of an increased excretion of calcium from the body. In 1970, Johnson and colleagues performed a study looking at the effects of protein intake on calcium excretion. They found that a high protein intake, particularly meat protein which has a high sulfur content, was responsible for an increased excretion of calcium from the body. Ingesting large amounts of protein actually increases the requirement for calcium. Other researchers, such as Linkswiler, Hegsted, Heaney, Walker, and their colleagues, have continued to confirm these conclusions.

In 1974, Mazess and Mather published a study that examined the bone-mineral mass of Eskimos on a high-meat diet and that of Caucasian omnivores on a comparatively low-meat diet. Again, the results revealed that the group consuming high amounts of meat had significantly lower bone mass

Considering Estrogen Replacement Therapy

The decision to start estrogen, or estrogen replacement therapy (ERT), is an important one that every woman who is approaching menopause or who is menopausal should consider. This is especially crucial if you have a high risk for osteoporosis. Current research shows that estrogen has a protective effect on preserving the bone mass in menopausal women. However, ERT isn't for everyone. Each woman must take her individual health profile and her family's medical history into account. For some women, the side effects and health risks either brought on or aggravated by ERT outweigh the benefits. The following chart lists the pros and cons.

Benefits of ERT	Possible Side Effects of ERT	Health Problems Aggravated by ERT
Reduced symptoms resulting from surgical menopause	Withdrawal bleeding	Previously diagnosed or suspected uterine endometrial cancer
Elimination of hot flashes and night sweats	Fluid retention	Previously diagnosed or suspected estrogen-dependent breast cancer
Decreased vaginal dryness, soreness, and pain during intercourse	Vaginal discharge	Liver and gallbladder disease
Reduced anxiety, irritability, mood swings, fatigue, and depression	Increased anxiety, irritability, moodiness	Hypertension
Improved skin and muscle tone	Headaches	Diabetes
Enhanced prevention or treatment of osteoporosis	Nausea	Uterine fibroid tumors
Enhanced prevention of heart attacks	Lower abdominal bloating	Endometriosis
Extended longevity	Estrogen allergy	Blood clotting

Some women prefer to address their menopausal symptoms naturally. Soy products have been found to aid in symptom relief. Soy
proteins contain plant estrogens that are potent enough to have an
impact on the body. New research is also showing that postmenopausal women who consume soy have healthier bones.

In addition to soy, there are a number of other natural ways
that women can prevent menopausal symptoms and preserve their
bone health. Some of these include dietary changes, vitamin/miner-
al supplementation, the use of herbs, stress reduction techniques,
and regular exercise.

than the group that consumed less meat. Researchers concluded that the
culprit was the meat protein in the diet.

In 1980, Marsh and colleagues published a study that cast further doubt
upon conventional approaches to the treatment of bone loss. The researchers recorded the effects of both vegetarian and omnivorous diets on bone
mass. The results of the study were astounding; the female meat-eaters had
a 35-percent loss of bone mass, while the vegetarian females only experienced an 18-percent loss of bone mass. These researchers concluded that
the differences in bone mass were likely the result of diet, and they target-
ed meat protein as the culprit.

Today, as research results continue to coincide with the above-dis-
cussed findings, health professionals are beginning to grasp the fact that
osteoporosis may be a disease that is due more to the excretion of calcium
rather than to its intake. If so, vegetarianism is certainly the better dietary
approach to follow.

Positive Effects of Soy-Protein Diets

Preliminary research on animals and humans have shown that soy may be
very instrumental in preventing osteoporosis and in helping the build-up of
bones. A study performed by Messina and colleagues and published in
1997 found that postmenopausal women who consumed a soy-based diet
had healthier bones than postmenopausal women who consumed a diet
with no soy or a moderate amount of soy. It is thought that soy's isoflavones—a particular family of phytochemicals (plant chemicals) that are
phytoestrogens—are considered to be especially beneficial to our health.

Vegetarians, especially vegans, tend to receive a lot of their protein
from soy and soy products. Perhaps this consumption of soy is giving them

the edge over their meat-eating contemporaries when it comes to bone health.

LOOKING AT LIFESTYLE

While some studies show no significant differences, many studies have found that vegetarians actually have greater bone density and lower incidences of osteoporosis than meat-eaters. Of course, researchers argue whether it is the abstinence from meat or the other lifestyle habits of vegetarians that give them the upper hand on stronger bones. Most likely, benefits come from both.

Importantly, physical activity—weight-bearing exercise, in particular—increases bone mineral density. The positive effects of exercise are enormous, influencing our physical, mental, and emotional being. Furthermore, smoking, alcohol, caffeine, and excessive salt consumption increase the excretion of calcium from the bones. Many people who are health conscious enough to follow vegetarianism are also health conscious enough to exercise regularly and to avoid harmful substances. As emphasized throughout this book, complete wellness in not achieved by observing one or two healthy habits. Health is achieved and maintained by making many health-promoting efforts. To assess whether or not you are at increased risk for osteoporosis, taking into acount your lifestyle habits, see "Checking Yourself: An Oseteoporosis Checklist," on page187.

PREVENTING OSTEOPOROSIS

Prevention will always be the best and most effective way to deal with osteoporosis. It behooves us to do our best to preserve our bones from an early age. The following summary of recommendations provides helpful guidelines:

- Minimize your calcium excretion by avoiding all of the following: meat protein; smoking; alcohol; caffeine; excessive salt.

- Engage in regular physical activity—walking, jogging, and lifting weights. Don't forget that weight-bearing exercises will increase your bone mass.

- Consume the suggested daily amounts of 1,000 to 1,300 milligrams of calcium and 5 to 15 micrograms of vitamin D. For a list of calcium-rich and vitamin D-rich vegan foods, see pages 236 and 244, respectively.

- Include plenty of soy and soy products in your diet.

Checking Yourself: An Osteoporosis Checklist

There are a number of factors that may place you at high risk for osteoporosis. Answer the following questions, checking the boxes for the questions to which you would answer "yes."

❑ Are you Caucasian or Asian (of Asian descent)?

❑ Do you consider yourself small-boned?

❑ Are you over 35 years of age?

❑ Do you have relatives who have had osteoporosis or frequent bone fractures?

❑ Do you do weight-bearing exercises less than three times a week?

❑ Do you smoke?

❑ Do you regularly take any of the following drugs, all of which interfere with calcium utilization: seizure control drugs; anti-inflammatory drugs; thyroid hormones (in large doses)?

❑ Have you ever been limited to bed rest for a prolonged period of time?

❑ Have you had zero full-term pregnancies?

❑ Do you follow restrictive diets for months at a time?

❑ Do you drink more than two alcoholic beverages per day? (1 drink: 12 ounces of beer; 4 ounces of wine; $1\frac{1}{2}$ ounces of hard liquor)

❑ Do you take large doses of vitamin A (over 5,000 IU/day) or vitamin D supplements (over 1,000 IU/day)? Overdosing on these vitamins can cause serious health complications (see page 68).

❏ Do you consume less than three servings of calcium-rich foods per day?

❏ Do you consume large amounts of meat?

❏ Does your diet consist of little, if any, soy or soyfood products?

If you answered "yes" to three or more of the above questions, you are at increased risk for osteoporosis. Talk with your health-care professional and take preventative measures.

If you follow these pointers, you will positively influence your bone health and your general health. Keep in mind that you do not want to overdose on calcium and vitamin D. Taking too much calcium can induce such symptoms as nausea, vomiting, high blood pressure, diarrhea, and constipation. An overload of vitamin D can also cause nausea and vomiting, in addition to loss of appetite, dry mouth, headache, fatigue, and dizziness. Furthermore, vitamin D toxicity can cause hypercalcemia, which is high blood-calcium levels that can result in irreversible calcium deposits in the organs and soft tissues of the body.

Osteoporosis is a widespread chronic disorder that especially afflicts women. Researchers and health professionals continue to argue over what the most effective approach to bone health is. Is it increased calcium intake, as most health professionals and the milk and dairy industry still claim? Or is it a diet that decreases the rate of calcium excretion from the body, such as a vegan diet? Despite these questions, one thing is for sure: vegetarians repeatedly have been found to have lower incidences of osteoporosis. And veganism, a diet which contains no animal protein, is an even safer bet.

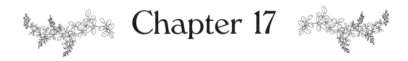

Chapter 17

Diabetes: Balancing Your Blood Sugar

At 5'5" tall, 45-year-old Diana Susek weighed 175 pounds. She was approximately 50 pounds overweight, despite her active lifestyle as wife, mother of three, and full-time working woman. Then Diana found out that she had high blood pressure and adult-onset diabetes. Diana's doctor started her on insulin and recommended that she see a dietitian for nutritional guidance, which she did. Although Diana was taking her insulin regularly and trying to follow her diet plan, she did not feel healthy.

Diana had been considering vegetarianism for a number of years, but didn't know if she could do it as a diabetic. Her dietitian did not promote it, so Diana began to research the available literature on diabetes and vegetarianism on her own. She found positive articles that encouraged her, and further support from health professionals who were more informed about vegetarian lifestyles. Diana decided to become a vegan. She now experiences more energy, greater peace of mind, and a general healthfulness that she hadn't felt since her youth. She has found that a vegan diet is a successful way to control her diabetes, her weight, and her high blood pressure.

When it comes to diseases that women fear, diabetes is probably near the bottom of the list. While the media bombards us with news of heart disease, cancer, and even osteoporosis, diabetes somehow tends to take a back seat. Don't let the lack of publicity fool you. Sixty percent of the newly diagnosed cases of diabetes are in women. In America alone, 6.5 million women suffer from this disease. It is a chronic illness that can lead to a number of serious health complications. So it is important that women learn how to prevent or manage diabetes. It is also important to realize that it is possible, even beneficial, to manage this chronic disease on a diet that avoids animal products. This chapter will discuss both the disease and the best ways to prevent it.

DEFINING DIABETES

In order to understand diabetes, we first must understand the regulation of sugar within our bodies. For proper functioning, it is necessary to maintain an adequate level of *glucose*—sugar in the blood. Glucose is the body's main energy nutrient; we need it in order to walk, run, talk, and even breathe. In essence, glucose is our fuel.

Most of what we eat can eventually be broken down into glucose. Carbohydrates are easily converted to this molecule, as they are simply strings of glucose molecules. Both fats and proteins also can be broken down into glucose. Fats are used before protein, since the body can store lots of fat and it is easier to convert it to glucose. Protein is usually broken down into glucose only in times of emergency, such as in the case of starvation.

Glucose is converted to energy within the cell. In order for glucose to get from the bloodstream into the cell, it needs a helper. This "designated driver" is *insulin,* which is a hormone produced by the pancreas. Every cell contains insulin receptors. If, for some reason, the body's cells do not readily accept the insulin (that is, if they become insulin resistant), or if there is no insulin to accept, glucose cannot enter into the cells and produce energy. In addition, glucose levels that are not properly regulated cause many health complications. This condition is known as *diabetes mellitus,* more commonly referred to as diabetes. The general risk factors for diabetes are heredity, obesity (and a high-fat diet), and aging.

There are two types of diabetes mellitus. The first kind is referred to as type I diabetes mellitus or insulin-dependent diabetes mellitus (IDDM). This disorder usually begins in childhood and is caused primarily by a viral infection that destroys the pancreas. When the pancreas is destroyed, the body's source of insulin is gone. Glucose cannot enter the cells and it accumulates in the bloodstream. Individuals who suffer from IDDM need to inject insulin directly into their bodies to remedy the problem.

Type II diabetes mellitus, or non-insulin-dependent diabetes mellitus (NIDDM), is more common; it is responsible for 85 to 90 percent of diabetic cases. A person with NIDDM *does* produce insulin—in fact, sometimes too much insulin—but the cells do not respond correctly to it. NIDDM is usually found in adults over 40 years of age and is strongly associated with obesity. Some scientists feel that when a person is obese, the excess fat actually interferes with the entrance of insulin into the cell.

There is another diabetic disorder called *diabetes insipidus*. It is not diet controlled, and therefore not applicable to our discussion on nutrition and vegetarianism. However, for a brief description of this disorder, see "A Different Type of Diabetes," below.

It is extremely important for people with diabetes mellitus to control their blood sugars effectively. The closer the blood sugars are to normal levels, the less complications that will occur. Poorly controlled diabetes is associated with numerous medical complications, including:

- atherosclerosis (plaquing of the arteries)

- damage to the eyes, resulting in impaired vision; diabetes is the leading cause of blindness in the United States

- damage to the nerves (termed *neuropathy)*, resulting in pain and/or loss of sensation in the limbs

- damage to the kidneys, causing kidney disease

- fifteen times higher risk of amputation due to gangrene

A Different Type of Diabetes

Scientifically speaking, "diabetes" refers to two different disorders: the more commonly recognized diabetes mellitus, and another disorder called diabetes insipidus. The latter is a disease that results from an inadequate production of vasopressin (a hormone), or the kidneys' incorrect response to this hormone. Vasopressin is responsible for keeping the body from producing too much urine.

Diabetes insipidus results in abnormal thirst and excessive amounts of urine. Urination is heavy at all times, even through the night and despite how much fluid is ingested. If an individual is losing too much liquid through frequent urination and is unable to restore the fluid balance of the body, she will become dangerously dehydrated. As a result, blood pressure drops and the body goes into shock. Taking vasopressin or a modified version of it into the body via nasal sprays, injections, or oral drugs treats this type of diabetes. The selected treatment will depend on the severity of the condition and the individual's health status.

- increased risk of infections, since bacteria thrive on sugar

- impaired circulation

A simple blood tests yields blood-glucose level. The normal range for blood-glucose is 70 to 120 milligrams per deciliter. Abnormally high blood-glucose concentration is referred to as *hyperglycemia*. It's characterized by many symptoms, including: acetone breath; confusion; dehydration; glucosuria (high concentration of glucose in the urine); intense thirst; labored breathing; nausea; and vomiting.

At the other end of the spectrum is low blood sugar, or *hypoglycemia*. This disorder is not necessarily associated with diabetes, but it is possible for a person with diabetes to become hypoglycemic—if a meal is skipped; if too much insulin or oral hypoglycemic medication is taken; or if strenuous exercise is performed without proper preparation. Symptoms of hypoglycemia include: dizziness; double vision; nervousness; shallow breathing; sweating; and weakness. The diabetic should always be prepared, in case of low blood sugar; she should have some type of quickly digestible sugar on hand at all times. Liquids are preferred above solids, as they can enter the bloodstream more rapidly. Sugar water, orange juice, and apple juice are excellent choices.

TREATING DIABETES

The goals of diabetic therapy are: to maintain blood-sugar levels within the normal range; to reduce weight, if necessary; and to allow the individual to continue with her routine duties and activities. The three main approaches to accomplishing these goals are: medications, including insulin and oral hypoglycemic agents; exercise; and diet. For information on diabetes during pregnancy, see "Diabetes Management During Pregnancy" on page 194.

Medications

Insulin is absolutely necessary for people with type I diabetes, since the pancreas is not producing any insulin. Oral hypoglycemic agents are used only for people with type II diabetes, and they work to stimulate the pancreas to secrete insulin. Actually, a person with type II diabetes may be given both insulin and oral hypoglycemic agents, but only if necessary, as a temporary or last resort. Many people with type II diabetes go on insulin for a brief while, and then lower the dose or get off insulin completely if they can manage their blood sugars well with exercise and diet.

Exercise

Exercise and diet are the primary modes of treatment for non-insulin-dependent diabetics. Exercise is crucial because regular physical activity contributes to weight loss, lowers the blood pressure, strengthens the cardiovascular system, and helps the individual to feel emotionally healthy too. Most importantly, exercise reduces the body's need for insulin, since it acts like insulin in helping the body to lower the blood sugars. Every person with diabetes who is able to exercise should be on a personal exercise regimen.

Dietary Habits

Diet is a vital component in treating non-insulin-dependent diabetes. Most people suffering from NIDDM are overweight or obese. Losing weight will enable them to maintain better control of their blood sugars, since it helps to lower the blood-glucose levels; the less a person weighs, the less insulin that is needed to maintain normal levels of glucose. So weight loss can actually result in lower medication doses.

For years, health professionals have told individuals with diabetes that they need to avoid all concentrated sweets, such as jellies/jams, cakes, cookies, sugar, honey, and molasses. The reason for this emphasis was due to the belief that concentrated sweets (or simple carbohydrates) do not need to be broken down extensively by the body. These simple sugars were thought to elevate the blood sugar immediately after eating, and then result in a large drop in blood sugar. On the other side, complex carbohydrates were believed to gradually increase and then decrease blood sugars, preventing quick changes. But recently, researchers have been finding that the effects of simple versus complex carbohydrates do not differ so significantly. Therefore, current diabetic guidelines have changed to include a small amount of concentrated sweets. However, on the whole, they still should be avoided not only because of their potential to raise the blood sugars, but also because most concentrated sweets are high in calories. Consuming excessive amounts of concentrated sweets is not considered a healthy eating practice for *any* individual.

Too much of anything can result in undesirable health problems. The individual with diabetes should give special consideration to the amount of foods eaten, not only for weight-control purposes, but also for blood-sugar-control purposes. Eating too much bread can raise your blood sugars to the same extent that a candy bar would. And eating three low-fat granola bars is just as bad as eating one that is high in fat. Portion sizes need to be

Diabetes Management During Pregnancy

Women with diabetes who are expecting to become pregnant and who are pregnant should realize that their disease places them at risk for several complications. The following is a list of complications that can occur:

- episodes of hypoglycemia and hyperglycemia

- spontaneous abortion (miscarriage)

- pregnancy-induced hypertension

- increased infant morbidity and mortality

- congenital abnormalities in the infant

Normal pregnancy in all females is characterized by an increase in blood-insulin levels and changes in insulin resistance. Insulin levels start to rise soon after conception, and they remain high. However, the tissues naturally become more insulin resistant. So women with diabetes need to closely monitor their blood-glucose levels and adjust their insulin dosages accordingly. The diet for pregnant women with diabetes is basically the same as the one for pregnant women in general, with one small change: consume a bedtime snack, to prevent hypoglycemia.

Gestational diabetes (GDM) is carbohydrate intolerance with an onset during pregnancy. It occurs when tissues become insulin resistant. One to three percent of all women who are pregnant will experience gestational diabetes. One-third of women who develop GDM will develop non-insulin-dependent diabetes within five years. It is very important to get screened for this disease because if it goes untreated, it is associated with a higher risk of infant and maternal illness, as well as infant mortality. The risk factors for gestational diabetes include: previous gestational diabetes; history of large infants (9 pounds or more); family history of diabetes; symptoms of diabetes and glucose in the urine; obesity and excessive weight gain; recurrent urinary tract infections; history of spontaneous abortions; and previously unexplained stillbirth(s). Dietary management of GDM is similar to non-insulin-dependent diabetes management for pregnant mothers.

controlled carefully. Acceptable portion sizes for the different vegan food groups are given in Table A.12, page 245.

Also, if you have diabetes—especially if you are on insulin or a hypoglycemic agent—be sure to eat your three meals at set times every day. Establishing regular hours for eating is important because it allows the body to get accustomed to a specific schedule. A light snack at night is also recommended, since blood sugars can dip very low in the night and you could wake up feeling very sick. Snacking between meals may be necessary, as well. You should speak with a dietitian for help in deciding the right amounts of food and the optimal times for eating.

BENEFITTING FROM VEGETARIANISM

Research has found that there is a lower incidence of diabetes among vegetarians. Most likely, this is because vegetarians tend to be leaner and closer to their ideal body weights than nonvegetarians. In addition, diabetes is less prevalent in people who consume high-fiber diets, and vegetarians generally consume a lot of fiber.

Here are a couple of research examples. A study on diabetes and nutrition, conducted by West and Kalbfleisch, looked at the prevalence of diabetes in eleven countries. Research results found that diabetes was associated with animal fat intake. Also, Snowdon and Phillips conducted a study on approximately 24,000 male and female Seventh-day Adventists aged 30 to 89 years of age. Some of the participants were vegetarian, while others were meat-eaters. Otherwise, the participants' lifestyles were very similar. The researchers found that a vegetarian diet was associated with a lower incidence of diabetes.

The incidence of diabetes among Seventh-day Adventists is 45 percent lower than the general population. As discussed throughout this book, the typical diet followed by Seventh-day Adventists is vegetarian and, therefore, high in fiber. A high-fiber diet is not only instrumental in promoting weight loss, but also has been found to improve glycemic control. So individuals with diabetes who are still consuming the standard American diet may improve their condition by following a vegetarian and, moreover, a vegan diet.

Meat, eggs, and dairy products are not necessary foods for anyone, let alone an individual with diabetes. As a matter of fact, a person with diabetes is at an increased risk for heart disease, so the low-saturated-fat, no-cholesterol vegan diet will not only help to improve glycemic control, but also to reduce the risk for developing heart disease in the future. A vegan who is diabetic can maintain her health and control her disease just as successfully, if not more successfully, than a meat-eater. Do not let uninformed individuals tell you otherwise.

PREVENTING DIABETES

As with other chronic illnesses, prevention is the best way to avoid the harmful effects of diabetes. Below are listed several suggestions for how to prevent this disease:

- Consume a diet that is high in complex carbohydrates and fiber, and limit your intake of saturated fats; the vegan diet will best fulfill these dietary guidelines.

- Achieve and maintain a healthy body weight.

- Engage in regular physical exercise; exercise improves glucose tolerance.

- Control/prevent hypertension (see Chapter 13).

- If pregnant, in order to reduce your risk of gestational diabetes, do not gain excessive weight.

Diabetes is another example of a disease that can be better managed, and perhaps prevented, through careful diet and exercise. As far as diet is concerned, a well-balanced vegetarian diet—especially the vegan diet—indeed can supply adequate nutrients, while providing lots of healthy fiber and little saturated fat and cholesterol. A vegan diet, in particular, will help control blood-sugar levels due to the high-fiber content, will contribute to weight loss if necessary, and will therefore aid in maintaining a healthy blood pressure.

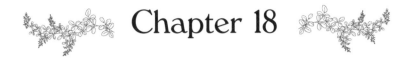

Chapter 18

More Reasons
to Go Meatless

Julie Morgan, a vegan of two years, was very excited when her mother stopped badgering her about her diet. To Julie's surprise, Mom started asking inquisitive questions such as, "What are the health benefits of eating a vegan diet?" and "Where did you get your information from?". The change of attitude came about because Julie's aunt died suddenly of a heart attack and, only a week later, her grandfather passed away from colon cancer. To top things off, Julie's dad was just diagnosed with gallstones.

Julie frequently discouraged her family from eating the traditional, high-fat, meat-based American diet. She is saddened that it took tragedy to get other family members to open their eyes to healthier eating options, but she is also excited that she can really start informing them about the benefits of vegetarianism now. Julie sets a wonderful example; her healthy energy and physical well-being attest to the fact that a vegetarian diet enhances life.

In addition to better prevention and better treatment of the chronic diseases discussed in Chapters 12 through 17, following a vegetarian diet gives you many more advantages. Read on for a few more ways in which your quality and possibly even duration of life can be enhanced through the vegetarian—better yet, vegan—lifestyle. As you will see, the benefits of becoming a vegetarian go on and on . . .

DIVERTICULAR DISEASE

The colon is lined with mucous membrane and surrounded by muscle. It is not uncommon for small areas of the mucous membrane to push out at places where there is weakness in the muscle. Tiny, pouch-like herniations, called diverticula, form. They are generally a result of constipation. In and of themselves, these diverticula should cause no problems. But if waste products lodge in them, infection and inflammation can result. This painful condition is termed *diverticulitis.* It is very common in Western countries such as the United States. The culprit is thought to be a low-fiber diet. Fiber makes feces softer and bulkier.

Diverticulitis can be symptomatic or asymptomatic, and chronic or acute. Millions of people have this condition, but many just attribute the symptoms—cramping; gas; bloating; abdominal tenderness on the left side; constipation; diarrhea; nausea; and frequent (almost constant) defeca-tion—to simple indigestion. The best way to prevent the condition is to fol-low a high-fiber diet and to drink a lot of water. Doctors instruct that if you are experiencing a diverticulitis attack, eat soft foods that will not require heavy work from your colon. Once the attack is over, strengthen your colon by eating bulk-promoting foods like fruit, whole grains, and raw vegeta-bles. Obviously, the vegetarian diet includes these health-promoting prac-tices by its very nature. So it has the advantage over the typical Western diet, again.

Mark Bricklin's *The Practical Encyclopedia of Natural Healing* con-firms that vegetarians are known to have less diverticular disease than meat-eaters. The book cites a study reported in the March 10, 1979 edition of *The Lancet.* The researchers of this study concluded that consuming more cereal fiber is responsible for the fewer cases of diverticulitis among vegetarians.

GALLBLADDER DISEASE

The gallbladder is a small organ that stores bile until it is secreted into the small intestines during digestion. Bile increases the solubility of fats, cho-lesterol, and vitamins in fatty foods, thus enabling our bodies to better absorb the nutrients. Gallbladder disease is not uncommon, and a Western diet—which, of course, includes meat—is one of the leading reasons why.

Diseases of the gallbladder include: *cholecystitis,* the inflammation of the gallbladder; *cholelithiasis,* the formation of gallstones in the gallblad-der; and *choledocholithiasis,* the obstruction of bile due to gallstones in the bile ducts. Normally, there is already a high content of liquid cholesterol in bile. If excessive amounts accumulate, the cholesterol may become insolu-ble, drain out of the bile, and form solid stones. The risk factors for choles-terol gallstones are: aging; diabetes; estrogen treatment; heredity; obesity (and high-fat diet); and pregnancy.

A greater number of women suffer from gallbladder disorders than men. The National Center for Health Statistics' *National Hospital Discharge Survey* approximates that 360,000 females had their gallbladders surgically removed in 1992 alone. It is important that women take dietary measures to decrease their risk. High-fat, low-fiber diets and obesity increase the risk of gallbladder disorders. A healthy vegan diet, which is naturally low in saturated fat and is high in fiber, can promote better gallbladder health.

The need for a cholecystectomy—the removal of the gallbladder— occurs more frequently in meat-eaters than in vegetarians. A study done by Pixley and colleagues investigated 762 British females. It found that the vegetarians in the group had a significantly lower history of cholecystectomies than the meat-eating participants. Furthermore, it was found that 17.8 percent of the meat-eaters had asymptomatic gallstones, as opposed to only 10.0 percent of the vegetarians.

A high intake of vitamin C has been found to decrease the risk of gallbladder disease. A review of this issue conducted by J.A. Simon found that vegetarian diets seem to protect individuals from the formation of gallstones because they are typically rich in vitamin C. Finally, a vegetarian diet may reduce the risk of gallstones simply by decreasing your risk of being obese and of getting diabetes, which are two major risk factors.

KIDNEY DISEASE

The kidneys take part in some of the most amazing functions of the body. They are recognized primarily for their role in excreting waste through the production of urine. However, these complicated organs are responsible for much more. They maintain fluid, electrolyte, and acid-base balance; help to regulate blood pressure; produce a hormone that stimulates the production of red blood cells; and activate vitamin D, thus aiding in the regulation of calcium level and bone metabolism.

Renal failure occurs when the kidneys are no longer able to perform the functions mentioned above. There are many possible causes for kidney disease and failure, but among them are some of the chronic illnesses that vegetarianism helps prevent and treat: atherosclerosis; hypertension; and diabetes.

Researcher Gretz and colleagues concluded that a vegetarian diet, especially one that includes soy, could help slow the progression of chronic renal failure. And D'Amico and his co-researchers published a study in 1992 reporting that people who suffer from nephrotic syndrome (kidney disorder) had a significant decrease in their urinary excretion of protein when they were placed on a soy-based vegetarian diet. This indicates better kidney function. Vegetarian diets can also benefit individuals with kidney disease who are at increased risk for heart disease because vegetarian diets are lower in saturated fat and cholesterol and can improve blood lipid levels.

If that's not enough, here's more evidence. High-protein diets are associated with hypertrophy (enlarging) of the kidneys and a decreased glomerular filtration rate (GFR). GFR is an indicator of kidney function. Such diets are also associated with the formation of kidney stones. In fact, one scientific review done by Goldfarb concluded that a high-protein intake was the most responsible factor in the development of kidney stones. A vegetarian diet is lower in protein than meat-based diets. Another study conducted by Ito and colleagues and published in 1992 found that individuals with calcium stones in their kidneys had significantly higher intakes of total protein and animal protein than the recommended guidelines. Furthermore, Marangella and fellow researchers compared healthy subjects with calcium-stone formers and determined that the calcium-stone formers should avoid excesses of animal proteins. Finally, a study published in 1988 reported that when Breslau's team of researchers assigned diets of equal protein to meat-eaters and vegetarians, they found that an animal-protein diet increased the risk of kidney stones. So a vegetarian diet is a smart decision when it comes to maintaining your kidneys at optimal health.

PERIMENOPAUSE

Hot flashes, night sweats, vaginal dryness, insomnia, and headaches are some of the symptoms associated with *perimenopause*—the time period before menopause when women experience changes in their estrogen levels. It's interesting to note that women from Japan rarely report experiencing the symptoms associated with perimenopause, while many American women suffer from them. Diet is thought to play a major role in this difference. The traditional Japanese diet is low in fat and rich in soy. In fact, the Japanese, as a population, consume the largest amounts of soy. You'll remember from previous discussions that soy contains phytoestrogens such as isoflavones. These specific plant chemicals have weak estrogenic effects.

Many females opt for estrogen replacement therapy (ERT) when they begin perimenopause and menopause. However, for some women, ERT has been associated with undesirable effects (see page 184). Females who include rich amounts of soy in their diets may be provided with the same benefits as those gained through estrogen replacement therapy, without putting themselves at risk for ERT's possible negative effects.

Vegetarians naturally consume more soy than meat-eaters, as soy is usually the main source of protein, as well as other nutrients, in the diet. Meat-eaters, on the other hand, often do not include soy at all in their diets, or they consume less of it. According to a study discussed in *The Soy Connection* (volume 5, number 1, 1997), the consumption of soyfoods providing at least 80 milligrams of isoflavones per day is associated with a reduction in the frequency of hot flashes. You can consume approximately 80 milligrams of isoflavones by eating two $\frac{1}{2}$-cup servings of tofu or other soyfoods. This is the amount recommended in the Daily Meal Pattern found in Chapter 4, page 47. For a list of isoflavone content in common soyfoods, see Appendix A, page 242.

PREMENSTRUAL SYNDROME (PMS)

Many of us suffer from discomfort—emotional and/or physical—for several days prior to menstruation. This condition has been termed *premenstrual syndrome (PMS)*. A woman with PMS can suffer from any number of the following symptoms: abdominal cramps; back pain; headaches; acne; swelling, soreness, and/or lumps in the breasts; water retention and resulting swelling; diarrhea; increased appetite; stronger cravings for sweets; thirst; and mood changes, ranging from nervousness to depression. In the *Encyclopedia of Natural Healing,* author Gursche makes a clear nutrition statement when discussing the symptoms of PMS: "A vegetarian diet is best. Vegetarians are more efficient than meat-eaters at excreting excess estrogen."

It has been found that vegan foods help some women find relief from PMS. In *365 Good Reasons to Be a Vegetarian,* Victor Parachin discusses a study on PMS conducted at the Massachusetts Institute of Technology. Judith Wurtman, PhD, placed premenstrual women on a high-carbohydrate, low-protein diet. In fact, the diet consisted of corn flakes with nondairy creamer. The results were striking; women who were grumpy and lethargic perked up, becoming pleasant and more alert. Wurtman proposes that a high intake of carbohydrates raises serotonin levels. Serotonin is a brain chemical that is involved in mood and sleep regulation. Nondairy products were used because milk protein actually reduces serotonin production. The conclusion was that a low-fat, low-protein, high-complex carbohydrate diet can relieve PMS symptoms. The vegetarian—especially the vegan—diet comes closest to meeting these criteria.

In *Menstrual Cramps: A Self-Help Program,* author Susan Lark, MD, offers dietary guidelines to help the reader. Lark explains the benefits of whole grains such as millet, rice, and oats; they provide considerable amounts of magnesium and calcium, which serve to relax muscle tension and naturally tranquilize our bodies. (However, avoid wheat because it contains gluten—a protein that is difficult to digest.) Whole grains also supply us with potassium, which acts as a diuretic, and fiber, which promotes healthy bowel movements and the excretion of excess fluid. Finally, whole grains offer B-complex and E vitamins, which give us an edge when it comes to fighting off fatigue and depression.

Lark also recommends an increased intake of legumes, vegetables, fruits, seeds, and nuts. Legumes supply us with calcium, magnesium, and potassium, as well as iron (which is needed during menstruation), copper, zinc, B-complex and B_6 vitamins, and fiber. Similarly, vegetables are often rich in calcium, magnesium, and potassium. Many also contain vitamin C, which fosters greater permeability of the capillaries, thus allowing more nutrients to enter the muscles and more waste to leave. Many fruits, too, contain vitamin C, calcium, magnesium, and, sometimes, fiber. And nuts and seeds add B-complex and vitamin E, magnesium, calcium, potassium, and the essential fatty acids to our diets. It is clear that vegan foods have the power to relieve PMS symptoms in a natural way.

Lark continues to suggest that very little or no meat be eaten. She explains that the body actually uses the saturated fats in red meats to produce chemicals that are responsible for the contraction of muscles and the constriction of blood vessels. Furthermore, Lark recommends the avoidance of dairy products, which also tend to result in muscle contraction. The salts in dairy can add to bloating and fluid retention. Tryptophan, found in dairy products, encourages drowsiness. This could be problematic when a female is already fatigued during her premenstrual and menstrual days. In addition, dairy has been found to decrease the amount of iron absorbed by anemic women; many females become anemic during menstruation. And a great number of us are allergic to milk products anyway. The typical allergic reactions—bloating, gas, bowel changes, cramps—can easily worsen symptoms of PMS. Finally, the saturated fats in dairy products and meat promote the production of too much estrogen, which can be responsible for fibroid tumors and, thus, more pain. The conclusion is simple: if you want to live a healthier, more comfortable life, follow a *vegan* diet. No one should subject themselves to unnecessary pain and agitation.

RHEUMATOID ARTHRITIS

The onset of rheumatoid arthritis can occur at any age, but it is more common in individuals 25 to 50 years old. It is a connective tissue disease causing an often painful inflammation of the joints, and usually affects several joints at once. Rheumatoid arthritis occurs more frequently in women; Susan Calvert Finn, in her article titled "Women in the New World Order: Where Old Values Command New Respect," asserts that 90 percent of people who suffer from rheumatoid arthritis are female.

According to *Overcoming the Pain of Inflammatory Arthritis: The Pain-Free Promise of Pantothenic Acid* by Phyllis Eisenstein and Samuel M. Scheiner, PhD, the symptoms of rheumatoid arthritis include: swelling; redness; stiffness; and warmth and tenderness upon touch. Eventually, the joints may become deformed and permanently stiff. In addition, other parts of the body become affected, thus leading scientists to consider rheumatoid arthritis a systemic disease and certainly an autoimmune disorder. Fleshy nodes may rise underneath the skin, commonly on the forearms and at the Achilles tendons. The eyes may become swollen and dry. Furthermore, the legs may be inflicted with sores that will not heal. Finally, lymph nodes may swell.

A few studies have been performed to observe the effects of a vegetarian diet on the symptoms of rheumatoid arthritis. For example, in his *365 Good Reasons to Be a Vegetarian*, Victor Parachin discusses a 1991 study performed by Dr. Jens Kjeldsen-Kragh of the Institute of Immunology and Rheumatology at the National Rheumatism Hospital of Oslo, Norway. The research showed that meatless diets resulted in relief from the symptoms of rheumatoid arthritis in nine out of ten patients. This relief included greater grip strength and significant reductions in pain, joint swelling, tenderness, and morning stiffness. The participants experienced improvement within one month. Furthermore, the improvement lasted throughout the study, which traced the subjects for an entire year. The researcher asserted that meat-eating exacerbates arthritis not only because of some people's allergic reaction to meat, but also because animal fat causes joint inflammation.

These findings have been confirmed by other research. In another study conducted by Kjeldsen-Kragh and colleagues and published in 1991, significant reductions in the number of tender and swollen joints, pain, and other symptoms were found when participants fasted for seven to ten days and then followed a vegetarian diet for one year. The fasting involved the consumption of only herbal teas, garlic, vegetable broth, decoction of potatoes and parsley, and juice extracts from carrots, beets, and celery. Kjeldsen-Kragh and co-researchers published yet another report in 1994, reporting that a group of subjects who responded well to a vegetarian diet continued to experience improved symptom control two years after the test diet was introduced.

Vegetarian diets, as well as many other food remedies such as watercress, burdock root, and alfalfa tea, have been disputed as effective against the treatment of arthritis. For example, a meatless diet is included in the American Dietetic Association's list of *unproven* regimens for arthritis. However, the research discussed in this section suggest otherwise. And in *Understanding Normal & Clinical Nutrition,* authors Whitney, Cataldo, and Rolfes report that research shows diets rich in fish oil EPA and low in saturated fats from red meats and dairy foods can help relieve the symptoms of arthritis. They also discuss the possible link between arthritis and poor immunity caused by diet.

As mentioned in Chapter 7, research showed that the incidence of arthritis was increased among women who had been overweight as teenagers. In *Understanding Normal & Clinical Nutrition,* the authors state that arthritis is identified as one of the consequences of obesity. They also go on to state, "Weight loss is important for overweight persons with arthritis, because the joints affected are often weight-bearing joints that are stressed and irritated by having to carry excess poundage." Vegetarians have a lower incidence of obesity, as proved by many studies. Vegetarianism can promote weight loss due to its low-fat, high-fiber content. Kjeldsen-Kragh and research colleagues, discussed on page 203, also reported that the study participants in the vegetarian diet group lost more weight than those in the control group.

SIGHT AND HEARING LOSS

In more than one way, it makes *sense* to follow a vegetarian diet. As Victor Parachin's *365 Good Reasons to Be a Vegetarian* explains, the vegetarian diet can promote better vision! Harvard researchers performed a study comparing participants who had age-related macular degeneration (AMD) with participants who did not suffer from the disease. AMD occurs when very small blood vessels grow behind a certain part of the retina, scarring and hemorrhaging result, and vision is impaired. The study concluded that the subjects who consumed the highest amounts of dark green, leafy vegetables, when compared with those who ate the least amounts, were 43-percent less likely to be afflicted with AMD.

Age-related macular degeneration is a prevalent and frightening problem, responsible for loss of vision in 13.1 million Americans. In fact, it is thought that AMD is the cause of at least one-third of the 900,000 cases of blindness in Americans. Why not play it safe and increase your intake of dark green, leafy vegetables? And what better way to make these dietary changes than to go vegan?

Sight isn't the only sense that will benefit from a vegan diet. It is now believed that hearing abilities are lower in areas where meat intake is higher. Again, according to Parachin, the hearing levels of residents of Moscow, Russia, where the average diet is high in animal products, were compared with the hearing levels of people living in the Georgian Republic, where the typical diet includes large amounts of plant foods. Both middle-aged and senior Georgians had higher hearing levels than the same age groups in Moscow. Interestingly, clerical workers who worked in a rather quiet environment in Moscow had poorer hearing than noise-exposed factory workers in Georgia. Researchers concluded that diet is apparently the responsible factor. Thus, it logically follows that a vegetarian diet would be of great benefit in keeping your hearing abilities at an optimal level.

As is evident throughout this chapter and all of Part Three, a vegetarian diet is associated with numerous health benefits and the prevention of a number of chronic diseases. If you are suffering from a particular illness, the information in these chapters is meant to encourage you toward healthier living, particularly through the observance of a vegan diet. However, you should seek the advice of a qualified health professional when deciding on treatment for any condition.

Part Four

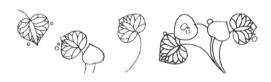

The Transition to a Plant-Based Diet

Becoming a successful vegan means trying new things, learning new ways, and creating a better life for yourself and others.

Chapter 19

Hints on How to Be a Successful Vegan

The more Elizabeth Wilson thought about it, the more she was convinced that the vegan diet would improve her health. It also fit right into her beliefs concerning compassion for animals and the preservation of the earth's resources. And she realized that veganism can help alleviate our world's hunger crisis. With all of this information constantly swirling through her mind every time she cooked chicken or downed a milkshake, Elizabeth finally decided to make the change. But tons of questions and concerns started to plague her mind day and night, causing her to second guess her decision: "What is the best thing to do first?" "Should I just cut the meat and dairy foods cold turkey, or should I do it gradually?" "How am I going to deal with my family?" Elizabeth needed to do some research—some reading and some talking. Accumulating knowledge is a necessary part of making the change to veganism.

It is time to engage in the wonderful process of becoming what I like to call a *successful vegan*. First, let me make one thing clear: being a vegan is both challenging and exciting. It is challenging in the sense that it involves a drastic change in your lifestyle, especially if you are a meat-eater. It is exciting because you are now embarking on a new way of life that promotes greater well-being in many ways. So, if you are presently considering veganism or if you've decided to become a vegan, Part Four of *The Vegetarian Female* is designed especially for you. This chapter will get you started with useful guidelines and tips.

HELPFUL HINTS ON MAKING THE TRANSITION

Different people are able to do different things. While some can quit a particular lifestyle habit—for example, smoking—quite easily, others have to go through a long and difficult process of unlearning an old habit, while learning new ones. Some will find that their lifestyles allow for change more easily than others; those who have families to feed or who are tight on time face special challenges when it comes to going vegan. Whatever your particular situation is, the following hints offer several key pointers as you begin your journey toward becoming a vegan.

1. Start out slowly. A gradual change gives both your body and your mind a chance to adapt to a new way of life. You might want to cut your portion sizes of meat in half, to decrease the number of days per week that you eat animal products, or to decrease the number of meals per day that you consume animal products.

2. Don't just abstain from foods; replace them. As you reduce your consumption of meat, eggs, and dairy, increase your intake of whole grains, beans, soyfoods, vegetables, fruits, and nuts.

3. Learn what vegan foods are rich in what nutrients. When you eliminate meat, dairy, and eggs, you most likely will be eliminating your main sources of such nutrients as protein, calcium, and iron. Appendix A will help you choose nutrient-rich vegan foods.

4. Plan your meals ahead of time. For example, plan a week of meals, incorporating your vegan goals. If you put some time aside to pre-arrange your meals, you will be more prone to actually accomplishing your goals because you will have taken into consideration the food items and preparation time necessary.

5. Don't be afraid to adjust the old recipes that you love most. Practically any dish can be made the vegan way. Today, there is a soy alternative for almost every dairy product and there are numerous meat analogs. Be brave—keep trying different products until you find ones that really work with your recipes.

6. Read labels. This will help you to identify products that contain ingredients you no longer want to include in your diet. Even foods like crackers, breads, and cold cereals often contain milk products. Familiarize yourself with the terms that manufacturers use on ingredi-

ent lists. For example, whey, calcium caseinate, and lactose refer to dairy products.

7. Ask a dietitian who is familiar with vegan meal planning to design a personal food guide for you. It should take into consideration your specific calorie, protein, and nutrient needs.

8. Keep a food diary for a couple of weeks, in order to keep track of your changing eating patterns and your progress.

9. If you eat out frequently, invest in *The Vegetarian Journal's Guide to Natural Foods Restaurants in the U.S. and Canada* (Avery Publishing Group, 1998). If you are planning to eat at a restaurant that is not specifically vegan/vegetarian, call ahead of time to find out if there are acceptable vegan options on the menu.

10. As you increase the amount of fiber in your diet, also increase the amount of fluid you drink.

HELPFUL HINTS ON KEEPING INFORMED

While you are making the transition to veganism, you will also need to learn a lot about nutrition. There is a wealth of information out there to support and guide you in your vegan lifestyle. Here are a few suggestions on accessing the latest nutrition news and gathering ideas for meals:

1. Subscribe to a vegetarian/vegan magazine, such as *Vegetarian Times.* See Appendix C for more information.

2. Become a member of a vegetarian/vegan support group in your community. You will find others who share your goals. Then you can set up a support network, as well as trade recipes and tips.

3. Learn to "surf the net" for interesting and new information about veganism. The internet has a number of helpful source sites. Appendix C lists several of them.

4. Check out the bookstore for new books on veganism and vegetarianism. As more and more people realize the benefits of a diet without animal products, more guidance and new ideas are being published.

5. Visit your local library and check out their selection of vegetarianism-based books, many of which will be helpful to the vegan. Talking with

your librarians may even alert them to collecting more literature on this subject.

HELPFUL HINTS ON DEALING WITH MEAT-EATERS

Worried about the upcoming holidays? What are you going to tell grandma when she prepares your once-favorite stuffed turkey? What are you going to do when you're invited to your best friend's annual Fourth of July barbecue? Or what about mom and dad berating you about your ridiculous decision not to eat a traditional Sunday breakfast anymore? First of all, remind yourself that there are hundreds, even thousands of vegans who have crossed these very same bridges and made it to the other side. Next, get prepared to defend your beliefs and to politely request to grill your own food. Here are a few helpful hints:

1. Be prepared with accurate information and a collection of winning facts. Therefore, you will feel confident and ready when you get those negative and inaccurate comments. A pamphlet containing a compilation of vegan-supporting facts from John Robbins' *Diet for a New America* is available for $1.00 through EarthSave Foundation, 706 Frederick Street, Santa Cruz, CA 95062–2205; telephone (408) 423–4069. Both the facts from John Robbins and *101 Reasons Why I'm a Vegetarian* by Pamela Teisler-Rice are also available over the World Wide Web.

2. Inform, *in advance,* whomever you will be eating with that you are a vegan, so that they are not shocked when you sit down to dinner. Yes, that means calling your aunt a week before Thanksgiving and filling her in on your lifestyle. Follow the news up with an offer to do #3, below.

3. Bring a vegan dish along when you are invited to eat at a meat-eater's house. This not only gives you an opportunity to eat a good meal yourself, but also a chance to win over some palates.

4. Never assume that people know what a vegan or a vegetarian does or doesn't eat. People's definitions of vegetarians range from those who exclusively eat plant foods to those who simply exclude red meat from their diets. Always be specific when explaining your eating habits.

5. Stand firm on your decision. The great majority of people have not researched the vegan lifestyle, and many will be too hard-headed to admit that you make good points. Stay calm and continue eating for life.

HELPFUL HINTS ON MOVING NONVEGANS TOWARD VEGANISM

There's no doubt that many moms and wives who have decided to become vegans are the only ones in their families willing to make such a healthy change. If this is the situation that you find yourself in, cooking according to your convictions may become a problem. How do you help move your meat-eating family toward veganism? Below are listed some helpful hints. Also, keep in mind that your family will probably be more open to going lacto-ovo- or lactovegetarian first, before going vegan. The gradual change is actually a good way to adjust the body and to break old habits in a healthy manner.

1. Identify plant foods that your family enjoys and prepare vegan dishes centered on those foods. If they love spinach, for example, try making tofu spinach patties or a spinach, chickpea, and rice dish.

2. Try mixing vegan products with meat in their favorite dishes. For instance, if they like a meaty spaghetti sauce or chili, use half of the meat you usually would and substitute the other half with meat analogs such as vegan crumbles or crumbled vegetarian burgers. If your family doesn't notice the difference, gradually make the replacement complete.

3. Reduce the frequency with which you prepare meat for your family. If your family is used to eating meat six days of the week, start serving meat on only five days of the week.

4. Reduce the portion sizes of meat. Add an extra vegetable or salad to make up for the change.

5. Since most individuals do not have a negative reaction to beans, nuts, vegetables, and fruits, start incorporating more of these foods in your family's diet. For example, prepare more bean-based soups and make available more vegetables and fruits as snacks.

6. Use soy-based cream cheese or sour cream for dips. Many people don't notice the difference.

7. Prepare a taste-tempting vegan dish that you think might win them over, such as barbecued tofu or sweet and sour tofu with vegetables.

8. Gradually educate your family, in a non-threatening manner, on the harmful effects of meat-eating and the benefits of veganism. Find a spe-

cific example of an individual whose diet has had a negative impact on his or her health and start discussing the importance of eating and living healthier.

9. Make a deal with your family. Tell them that you are trying to become a vegan and would appreciate their support, and also explain that you are concerned about their health as well. Inform them that one or two nights per week, you will be preparing an all-vegan meal. Give them a couple of vegan/vegetarian cookbooks to look through, and let them have some input on what meals will be prepared.

10. Tell your family that you are treating them to dinner. Then take them out to a vegetarian restaurant, or encourage them to choose a vegetarian meal at a nonvegetarian restaurant. Chinese and Italian restaurants usually have good vegetarian choices.

You must remember that change is vital to life. From the time we are born to the time we die, our bodies, minds, and every aspect of our humanity are involved in change. We go from breastmilk to soft foods, to finger foods, to cups, forks, and spoons. We go from a flat chest to a well-developed female figure. (Well, at least some of us do.) We go from being squeamish about relationships to seeking profound love. Change is beautiful, as long as we make sure that we are changing for the better and not for the worse.

A healthier body is what the change to veganism means. It is about reducing your family's risk of such diseases and conditions as heart disease, cancer, and obesity. It is about meeting your nutritional needs on a diet that is aimed at preserving and protecting our environment, our animals, and ourselves. It is about enhancing life and enjoying nature's bounty.

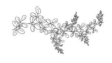

Chapter 20

Purchasing, Storing, and Preparing Vegan Foods

Two months after she had made the decision to go vegan, Patricia Glavic found herself having a difficult time. She was not familiar with many of the vegan foods and did not know how to prepare them. She could not find many soy products in her local grocery store. Her frustration grew every day. What Patricia needed was a beginner's guide, so to speak.

Patricia turned to researching the basic facts on maintaining a vegan diet—tips on buying and storing food, product names of meat and dairy alternatives, and suggestions on good cookbooks to provide a number of delicious dishes. She soon found herself becoming an expert shopper of health foods and an innovative cook. It didn't happen overnight, but now living as a vegan comes naturally and simply to Patricia.

The difficulties that Patricia faced are common ones; perhaps you are going through a similar experience. At first, purchasing and cooking vegan foods can be intimidating—you may feel as though your choices are very limited. But the longer you practice veganism, the easier it will get. To get you off to a great start, this chapter will offer you basic guidelines for purchasing, storing, and preparing vegan foods.

WHOLE GRAINS AND STARCHES

There is a variety of grains with which to familiarize yourself. These grains come in many different forms. The groats—grain kernels with the outer hull removed—are usually used for hot cereals, while the flours serve as the main ingredients for baking bread and for making pasta and other delights. Table 20.1 provides a list of grains and the different forms in

20.1. Whole Grains and Their Available Forms

Whole Grain	Available Forms
Amaranth	Seeds; flour
Barley	Hulled; pearled; flour
Buckwheat	Groats; kasha; flour
Corn	Hominy grits; meal; flour
Millet	Groats; couscous; meal; flour
Oats	Groats; steel-cut; rolled; quick; flour; bran
Quinoa	Seeds; flour
Rice	Long/short grain; brown; white wild; bismuth arboria; flour
Rye	Berries; flakes; flour
Wheat	Whole; berries; cracked; bulgur; couscous; flakes; flour; gluten flour; stone ground flour; wheat germ

which they are available. Grains are a very important part of the vegan diet. In fact, this food group should start your day. See "Grains in the Morning, on page 217.

Purchasing Cereals and Other Starches

Your local grocery store probably carries only a few grain products, including bleached and unbleached wheat flour, whole wheat flour, corn meal, and quick oats. These items are inexpensive. The other grain products mentioned above, such as bran couscous and hulled barley, are available in most health food stores. These products will be more expensive because they are more difficult to obtain and have a low demand.

Breads also fall into the category of grains and starches. For information on this type of food, see the inset titled "Vegan Breads," on page 219.

Storing Cereals and Other Starches

Generally, cereals and other starches can be stored for long periods of time. Extensively prolonged storage—for example, years—promotes the development of little bugs called weables. So store your starch products in airtight containers.

Grains in the Morning

Breakfast is one of the most important and most frequently missed meals of the day. Whole grain cereals/starches, by far the most widely used foods throughout the world, should be a component of your breakfast. Among the healthy hot, cooked cereal choices are oatmeal, *Wheatena*, corn meal mush, and *Cream of Wheat with Wheat Germ*. Suggested cold, ready-to-eat cereals are General Mills' *Whole Grain Total*, Kellogg's *Wheat Total*, and *Kellogg's Product 19*, *Cheerios*, and *Musleux*.

Preparing Cereals and Other Starches

Most cereal grains and other starches need to be cooked in order to be eaten. The majority of grains are cooked by boiling them in water in a pot over high heat. Once they boil, you generally decrease the heat to a "low" setting and cover the grains, allowing them to simmer for a set time.

Cooking times vary according to the type of grain or cereal. Whole grains take longer to cook than processed grains. For example, brown rice has a longer cooking time than white rice. You can further soften grains by cooking them in more water for longer periods of time. Less water renders a firmer texture. For cooking times on several types of grain, see Table 20.2. The information is taken from Sandra Woodruff's *Secrets of Cooking for Long Life*. Woodruff also explains that cooking time can be halved for those grains that take exceptionally long times—for example, barley and brown rice—by soaking the grains overnight or for eight hours.

Some people find that starches taste bland. Therefore, they like to add salt to their starch dishes. Don't forget that there are plenty of other seasonings that can add flavor such as low-sodium taco seasoning for a Spanish flair. It is a good idea to start out with a light hand and add more herbs or spices as your taste desires.

FRUITS AND VEGETABLES

It seems a constant challenge to preserve the texture, color, flavor, and, most importantly, the nutrient content of fruits and vegetables. Fresh fruits and vegetables have been hailed as offering superior nutrition. Growing your own produce allows you to cut the time that it takes for the produce to reach your table. The fresher the produce, the tastier, better looking, and

Table 20.2. Cooking Grains		
Grain (1 cup)	**Amount of Water**	**Cooking Time**
Barley (hulled/pearled)	$2\frac{1}{2}$ cups	50–60 min
Brown rice	$2\frac{1}{2}$ cups	45–50 min
Buckwheat (groats/kasha)	$2\frac{1}{2}$ cups	15–20 min
Millet	3 cups	20 min
Oats, old-fashioned	2 cups	5–20 min (stir occasionally)
Oats, quick	$1\frac{3}{4}$ cups	1 min
Quinoa	2 cups	10–15 min
Rye, cracked	$2\frac{1}{2}$ cups	15–20 min
Rye, rolled	2 cups	20 min
Wheat, bulgur	$1\frac{1}{2}$–2 cups	*Special instructions:* In large, heatproof bowl, pour boiling water over bulgur; stir, cover, let stand for approximately 30–45 min
Wheat, cracked	$2\frac{1}{2}$ cups	15–20 min
Wheat, rolled	2 cups	20 min
Wild rice	$2\frac{1}{2}$ cups	50–60 min

more nutrient-dense it is. However, not all of us have the time and/or the property to grow our own produce. Below are some helpful suggestions on what the next best options are.

Purchasing Fruits and Vegetables

Depending on where you live, you might find the purchasing of fruits and vegetables to be more expensive than you would like, especially the more exotic and ethnic varieties like plantains, chayote, collard/turnip/mustard greens, kiwis, starfruit, and mangoes. In addition, you may be unable to find much variety in your local grocery stores. I was able to overcome both the expense and the variety problems by finding an open market known as

Vegan Breads

Nothing can compare with a slice of warm homemade bread with your favorite spread. Only homemade bread gives you that special texture, taste, and aroma. Baking bread does not have to keep you in the kitchen all day; it is probably easier than you think. Eggs and milk are not necessary to produce a beautiful loaf of bread; you can use basically any bread recipe you desire and simply eliminate the eggs and dairy products. No substitution is necessary. This is also true for muffins. Regarding butter or lard in these recipes, I substitute with margarine or oil. Vegetable shortening is another alternative.

For those of us who simply cannot find the time or the skill for homemade bread, there are a few available vegan breads at the grocery store. Whole wheat and whole grain breads cost more than breads made with bleached/unbleached wheat flour. Make sure that you read the ingredient list to confirm that the bread you are buying is a vegan loaf.

Both freshly baked and store-bought bread should be used within the week. It is best to keep bread in airtight boxes or bags. Also, refrigeration helps to keep it fresh.

the West Side Market in Cleveland, Ohio. There might be a similar market that offers more variety for less money in your neck of the woods, too. You'd be surprised what you'll find out just by asking around.

In most states, the summer months are the months that cater to gardening. I found that I live near several gardeners who sell their fresh produce at extremely reasonable prices. The benefits do not just end or begin with the price, however. The local gardeners' fresh produce looks better and larger, as well as tastes fresher and more flavorful, than the store-bought produce. And local farmers/gardeners often do not use the high amount of pesticides that commercial farmers use. So if you do not have a green thumb or, for whatever reason, can't garden, go searching for some local gardeners who are selling their fruits and vegetables. You won't regret it.

Another way to obtain fresh produce is to ask your grocer the delivery date for fresh fruits and vegetables. And if you're watching your pocketbook, keep in mind that purchasing in-season produce is less expensive than out-of-season produce. You will, however, have to sacrifice variety somewhat if you stick to seasonal fruits and vegetables. Finally, you might find usable produce on the discount rack. The produce may not be the freshest, but it can still serve a purpose, especially if you are seeking produce to use in baking or canning or for immediate use. Bananas are a good example, since they usually go on the discount rack when those brown spots appear. Actually, that's the best time to eat them, for they are truly ripe in their grape-sugar stage. Spotted bananas make delicious banana bread, too.

Of course, there are other options to fresh produce, such as frozen fruits and vegetables. You might have heard that frozen vegetables are the healthiest choice, since the freezing climate preserves more of the nutrients than the open air. In truth, the longer the produce sits—at no matter what temperature—the more nutrients that are lost. However, frozen fruits and vegetables are certainly better than canned. Sometimes they're even better than fresh. For example, frozen collards contain more vitamin C and calcium than fresh collards.

Canned fruits and vegetables are the least desirable type of produce to purchase. The canning process involves cutting the fruit or vegetable up into appropriately sized pieces. This allows more of the produce to be exposed to the air and, thus, more nutrients are lost. In the case of fruits, canning involves removing most of the fibrous portions, such as the skin. In the case of vegetables, the produce is thoroughly cooked. When we open a can, we need to reheat the vegetables, causing a further loss of nutrients. Canning also involves the addition of juices or sauces that are usually high in salt and sugar.

Canned fruits and vegetables do have their advantages though, especially when it comes to shelf life. And most of today's manufacturers do add back some of the nutrients that have been lost in the processing. In many cases, canning companies add nutrients during the canning process; this provides some supplementation.

Dried fruits have many advantages. First, they are more nutrient-dense per serving than other packaged fruits. And they have a long shelf life. Your local health food store should offer a wide variety of dried fruits.

Storing Fruits and Vegetables

Fresh fruits and vegetables should not be stored for long periods of time, as nutrition is compromised with time. Most are best stored in the refrigerator for no more than a week. Some produce, such as tomatoes, should be stored outside of the refrigerator.

Freezing your fruits or vegetables is a good alternative when you want to increase their storage life. For example, freezing allows you to keep greens for a week or two, rather than for a day or two. If you cannot get to the market weekly to shop for fruits and vegetables, buying frozen vegetables or freezing your vegetables is a good idea. Canned vegetables and fruits have an extremely long shelf life. But remember, much of the produce's nutritional content is lost in the canning process. Finally, if you keep dried fruits well wrapped/packaged, they will last quite a while.

Preparing Fruits and Vegetables

The preservation of the nutrients greatly depends on how you choose to prepare/cook the foods. One of the first rules to always consider in preparing produce is: *only cook that which cannot be eaten raw.* Raw food is, by far, more nutritious than any type of cooked food.

One of the nicest things about fruits is that all you need to do is wash and eat. Vegetables, on the other hand, are not always eaten raw. When cooking vegetables, there are some ways to avoid unnecessary vitamin loss. First, do not pre-cut vegetables, since that provides increased air exposure. Cutting of vegetables should be done immediately before cooking. Then, cook your vegetables at lower temperatures. This decreases the amount of vitamin destruction. Also, use as little water as possible when cooking vegetables. Most vegetables do not need any water added if they are cooked on a low fire.

Do not overcook vegetables. If you are just learning how to cook certain types, a helpful resource is Marion Bennion's *Introductory Foods.* Bennion offers basic guidance for cooking commonly eaten vegetables like broccoli, carrots, and onions, as well as for cooking less "mainstream" vegetables like artichokes, beet greens, rutabagas, and turnip greens. Table 20.3 gives some examples of cooking times, as suggested by *Introductory Foods.* Pressure cooking instructions apply to 15 pounds of pressure.

Baking, steaming, panning, and stir-frying are the best cooking methods to use; frying and boiling cause greater nutrient loss. In addition, learn to portion the amounts that you cook, so that you can avoid having leftover vegetables. Leftovers involve storing time and reheating, causing further nutritional loss. Finally, serve vegetables immediately after cooking. Holding them aside increases nutrient loss.

Of course, seasoning is a wonderful part of preparing vegetable meals. Onions, bell peppers, garlic, seasoning salt, low-sodium soy sauce, basil, *Mrs. Dash*; and *Washington's Vegetable Seasoning* packets add exciting flavor to almost any vegetable dish.

Table 20.3. Cooking Vegetables

Vegetable	Amount of Water	Cooking Time
Broccoli (1½–2 lbs)	*Boil:* enough to cover	*Boil:* flowerets, 5–10 min; stems, 10–15 min
	Pressure cook: ⅓ cup	*Pressure cook:* 1½–2 min
Brussels sprouts (¾ to 1 qt)	*Boil:* enough to partially cover	*Boil:* 10–15 min
	Pressure cook: ½ cup	*Pressure cook:* 1–2 min
Cabbage (1 lb)	*Boil:* enough to partially cover	*Boil:* 6–9 min Steam: 9–10 min
	Pressure cook: ½ cup	*Pressure cook:* young cabbage, 1–1½ min; mature cabbage, 2–3 min
Corn, young green, on the cob	*Boil:* enough to cover ears	*Boil:* 5–10 min Steam: 10–15 min
	Pressure cook: ½ cup	*Pressure cook:* 1–2 min
Potatoes, Irish (1–1½ lbs)	*Boil:* for whole, enough to barely cover; for cut, enough to partially cover	*Boil:* whole, 30–35 min; cut, 20–30 min Steam: whole, 40 min; cut 30–35 min Bake: whole, 40–60 min;
	Pressure cook: for whole, 1 cup; for cut, ¾ cup	*Pressure cook:* whole, 15 min; cut, 8 min
Potatoes, Sweet (1–1½ lbs, whole)	*Boil:* enough to barely cover	*Boil:* 30–35 min Steam: 35–40 min Bake: 30–50 min
	Pressure cook: 1 cup	*Pressure cook:* 8–10 min
Turnips (1 lb)	*Boil:* enough to partially cover	*Boil:* 15–20 min Steam: 20–25 min
	Pressure cook: ½ cup	*Pressure cook:* 1½–4 min

LEGUMES

Legumes—or beans, as they are more commonly known—are highly nutritious and promote balance within your meals. There are many varieties of legumes; see Table 20.4 on page 224. The information is from *The Instant Bean* by Sally and Martin Stone. Legumes can be prepared as a main dish or as a side dish. They are great in soups and dips. They liven up pasta and salad entrées. It seems that the possibilities are endless. One book that can get you started on learning how to prepare beans in a variety of ways is *Bean Banquets from Boston to Bombay* by Patricia Gregory (Woodbridge Press Publishing, 1983).

Purchasing Legumes

Many legumes are readily available in your local grocery store. They are rather inexpensive. In fact, legumes are probably one of the least costly food items that go such a long way in terms of nutrition and storage life. Some legumes, such as soybeans, might not be available at your grocery store, but you should find them at your local health food store.

Canned legumes are quick alternatives. Chickpeas, red beans, vegetarian chili, and vegetarian refried beans are commonly canned legumes and are available at any grocery store.

Storing Legumes

Legumes can be stored for long periods of time. My family has kept beans for years. Since they are dried, they do not spoil and they do not go rancid. However, the longer you store them, the longer they take to cook. Plastic or glass containers are ideal for storing legumes. You can also freeze cooked beans. They can last months in the freezer.

Preparing Legumes

It is necessary to cook legumes before eating them, since cooking improves their flavor, makes them softer and more digestible, and destroys some potentially toxic substances. Legumes, or beans, generally take a significant amount of time to cook, which is probably one of the reasons that they are not readily consumed by most people. Knowing when to start cooking legumes and learning the different ways to cook them can make your daily preparation of beans simple and hassle-free.

In preparing your beans for cooking, they should be picked and rinsed. Bad beans and dirt might be mixed in with the good beans. Ideally, beans should be soaked overnight; if that's not possible, soaking them for an hour or two may be enough to do the trick. Soaking the legumes softens them, allows them to rehydrate, and reduces their cooking time. Some types, such as split peas and lentils, do not need to be soaked. See Table 20.4 on page 224 for more information.

Table 20.4. Approximate Soaking and Cooking Times for Legumes

Type of Bean	Soaking Time	Stove-top Cooking	Pressure Cooker
Adzuki	4 hr	1 hr	15 min
Black Beans	4 hr	1 hr, 15 min	15 min
Black-eyed Peas	—	30 min	—
Lima Beans	4 hr	1 to $1\frac{1}{2}$ hr	20 min
Cannellini	4 hr	1 hr	15 min
Chickpeas	4 hr	2 to $2\frac{1}{2}$ hr	25 min
Dals	—	25 min	—
Fava (Broad Beans)	12 hr	3 hr	40 min
Ful Nabed (Broad)	12 hr	3 hr	40 min
Great Northern	4 hr	1 hr	15 min
Brown Lentils	—	25 min	—
Green Lentils	—	30 min	—
Red Lentils	—	20 min	—
Mung Beans	4 hr	45 min to 1 hr	—
Split Peas	—	30 min	—
Whole Peas	4 hr	40 min	15 min
Pigeon Peas	—	25 min	—
Mexican Beans (Pink, Calico, Red)	4 hr	1 hr	20 min
Pinto Beans	4 hr	1 to $1\frac{1}{2}$ hr	20 min
Red Kidney Beans	4 hr	1 hr	20 min
White Kidney Beans	4 hr	1 hr	20 min
Small Navy Beans	4 hr	2 hr	25 min
Soybeans	12 hr	3 to $3\frac{1}{2}$ hr	30 min

After soaking, legumes should be rinsed; oligosaccharides, which are the culprits of gas associated with bean consumption, can cling to them. Throw out the soaking water and place them in fresh water before cooking.

Three ways to cook legumes are discussed below. Notice how cooking time changes according to method.

Electric or Gas Stove. When cooking beans on the stove, it is best to cover them and to use a low to moderate fire. Table 20.4 gives stove-top cooking times for some popular beans, as recommended in Sally and Martin Stone's *The Instant Bean.* Of course, if you do not soak the dried beans, cooking time will be longer.

Pressure Cooker. When using a pressure cooker for your legumes, use a ratio of 1 cup of beans to 3 cups of water. Place the top of the pressure cooker on, and make sure that the cover is fitted properly and perfectly sealed. Bring the legumes to a high pressure for 5 minutes and then let the pressure fall. Next, bring them back to a high pressure for the length of time required to cook the beans. Pressure cooking greatly reduces cooking time. Again, see Table 20.4 for more information. The pressure-cooking instructions apply to the use of 13 pounds of pressure. Again, if the beans have not been soaked, cooking time will be longer.

Crock Pot. Using a crock pot is one of the simplest ways to cook beans. This method requires longer cooking time—generally double or triple the time to cook when compared with other methods—but causes the least hassle. While the beans gently and slowly cook in the crock pot, you can go to work or go to bed at night. (I usually cook them the day before I need to use them.) Place the legumes in the crock pot in a ratio of 1 cup of beans to 3 cups of water. Turn the crock pot on and let the legumes cook. Check for doneness; they are ready to eat simply when their softness is to your liking.

You can increase the flavor of bean dishes by adding some simple seasoning. I suggest adding one or more of the following: chili powder; tomato sauce; garlic powder; salt; basil; onion powder; fresh onions and garlic; a touch of sugar; *Washington's Vegetable/Onion/Brown/Golden Seasoning;* and vegetarian bullion seasonings.

Let's face it. For most of us, it's not the buying, storing, or preparing of beans that is the greatest worry. Instead, it's the unpleasant gas that follows. Thankfully, *Beano* is available on the market today. This product helps to eliminate, or at least reduce, this undesirable aftereffect.

MEAT AND DAIRY ALTERNATIVES

There are several different types of meat and dairy alternatives available in the market place today. They range from frozen tofu hot dogs to canned chili beans. Most are made from texturized vegetable/soy protein and tofu. Meat and dairy alternatives can add tremendous variety to your meals. Vegan luncheon slices or garden burgers make delicious sandwiches. (Smear on some *Veganaise* or *Nayo,* great substitutes for regular mayonnaise.) And vegan hot dogs grill just as nicely as regular hot dogs. Table 20.5 lists a number of meat and dairy alternatives, suggests brands, and explains what nonvegan foods they can replace.

Purchasing Meat and Dairy Alternatives

Most meat alternatives are not found in your regular grocery store. A health food store is the primary place where many of the above-named products can be found. Vegetarian meat alternatives are expensive, but they are not essential to being a vegan. Some vegetarians use these items only on special occasions, when they want something a little different or when they want something to grill. Others make them a regular part of their diet. Still others do not rely on them at all. The Soy Foods Directory is an excellent resource that lists soy companies and their soy products, including many meat and dairy alternatives. See Appendix C on page 251 for information on this directory, so that you can order your free copy.

Storing Meat and Dairy Alternatives

Most meat and dairy alternatives come either canned or frozen and, thus, can be stored for long periods of time. There are usually expiration dates printed on the packages.

Preparing Meat and Dairy Alternatives

Most meat alternatives can be prepared as you would prepare the actual meat products. For example, a *Tuno* sandwich is made in the same way as a tuna sandwich (but substitute mayo with *Nayo* or *Vegannaise*). But you usually don't have to "cook" the meat alternatives; just heat them. Most products contain recipes on the packages.

NUTS AND SEEDS

Though the recommended serving size of nuts and seeds—usually 1 ounce—is not very big, this food group packs in a lot of nutrition. Here is a list of nuts and seeds that you can add to your diet:

- almonds
- Brazil nuts
- butternuts
- cashews
- chestnuts
- coconuts
- filberts/hazel nuts
- hickory nuts
- macadamia nuts
- peanuts
- pecans
- pine nuts
- pistachios
- pumpkin seeds
- sesame seeds
- sunflower seeds
- walnuts

Purchasing Nuts and Seeds

The most expensive vegan food is nuts, yet they are also one of the most nutritious. Most grocery stores do not stock raw nuts and seeds, which are preferable, but health food stores do. The grocery stores will carry commercial brands of nuts like *Eagle* or *Planters*. Often, commercial-brand nuts are baked and have additional oil added.

Storing Seeds and Nuts

Because of their fat content, nuts and seeds can go rancid in a few weeks. Shelled nuts should be stored in plastic bags with holes, tightly sealed tin cans lined with paper, or frozen. Unshelled nuts last a lot longer; most unshelled nuts can be stored in plastic bags/containers in the refrigerator or freezer for up to a year.

Preparing Nuts and Seeds

Nuts and seeds are best when eaten raw, especially since most brands add a lot of oil and salt during the roasting process. Or by learning to roast your own nuts, you can control the amount of added salt and fat.

Most of us just pop nuts into our mouths like popcorn, and that is a great way to eat them. You can also sprinkle ground nuts or seeds on top of foods such as cereals and fruit salads. Or add ground nuts or seeds to baked foods such as cookies, vegan meatloaf, and bread. How about using nuts and seeds in dishes like stir-fried vegetables, rice, and salads? Also, consider replacing your margarine or butter with nutbutters. You can make and use nut milks, such as almond milk, for cereal and other foods. Finally, make a snack dish that includes nuts and seeds—mix them with raisins or make a party mix.

Table 20.5. Vegan Alternatives to Meat and Dairy Items

Food Item	Suggested Brand/Product	Uses
Breakfast patties; links	*Green Giant; Loma Linda's Little Links and Linkets*	As a substitute for meat sausages/links; in sandwiches
Chili beans (canned)	*Chili Man; Health Valley Chili; Worthington and Low Fat Chili; Nature Touch Vegetarian Chili*	In sandwiches such as chilidogs; on rice; with chips and salsa
Cream cheese alternative	*Tofutti's Better Than Cream Cheese*	As a substitute for cream cheese
Ice cream, dairyless	*Tofutti; Rice Dream*	As a substitute for ice cream
Luncheon slices (refrigerated)	*Veggie Cuisine (YVES); Lightlife*	In sandwiches; on relish trays
Milk alternatives	*Solait; Rice Moo; Fearn Soya Powder; Naturally Almond; Rice Dream; West Soy Plus and Non-Fat; EdenSoy*	As a substitute for milk, with cereal; in recipes; by the glass; etc.
Sour cream alternatives	*Soymage; Tofutti*	As a substitute for sour cream, in baked goods and dips, and as a spread
Soy cheese	*Soymage*	As a substitute for cheese, in sandwiches and in recipes
Soy protein log (frozen texturized)	*Worthington's Chickets*	Diced in salads; sliced in sandwiches; breaded and baked/fried; etc.
Tofu, firm non-silken	*NaSoya; White Wave; Spring Creek;* local tofu (for example, Cleveland tofu)	As a substitute for scrambled eggs, and baked, fried, and shish-kabob meats; in salads—pasta, potato, tossed; in rice; with stir-fry veggies

Table 20.5. Vegan Alternatives to Meat and Dairy Items (cont.)

Food Item	Suggested Brand/Product	Uses
Tofu, silken	*Mori Nu Silken Tofu* (soft/medium/ firm/low fat)	In tofunnaise, puddings, sauces, salad dressings, and shish-kabobs
Tuna substitute (frozen log and canned)	*Worthington's Tuno*	In pasta salads, casseroles, sandwiches, and dips
Turkey roll alternative	*Worthington*	In sandwiches, salads; sliced, with vegan gravy
TVP (texturized vegetable protein; must be rehydrated)	Local brands of soy chunks, granules, and strips	Chunks and strips: in soups and stews, or as rice/pasta toppers; granules: to sustitute for ground beef in recipes
Vegan burger crumbles; texturized vegetable/ soy protein	*Light Life's Meatless Gimme Lean; Nature Touch; Green Giant; Morningstar*	In spaghetti sauce, to replace chopped meat; as a substitute for meat in meatballs, sandwiches, tacos and burritos; in veggie-burgers, veggie-loaves, and veggie-patties
Vegan burgers (frozen)	*Morningstar's Fat Free Better-N-Burgers; Green Giant; Nature Touch; Lightlife; Mudpie*	In sandwiches; crumbled in spaghetti sauce
Vegan dinner cuts/ choplets/cutlets (canned)	*Countrylife; Loma Linda's Dinner Cuts; Worthington's Low Fat Choplets; Worthington's Low Fat Multigrain Cutlets*	In sandwiches, breaded and fried/baked

Table 20.5. Vegan Alternatives to Meat and Dairy Items (cont.)

Food Item	Suggested Brand/Product	Uses
Vegan mayonnaise	Veganaise; Vitasoy's NaSoya Nayonaise	As a dressing on salads and sandwiches
Vegan scallops (canned)	Worthington's Low Fat Skallops	In stews; breaded and fried/baked
Vegan steaks (canned)	Worthington	Breaded and fried/baked; in sandwiches
Vegetarian burgers (canned)	Loma Linda's	In spaghetti sauce; as a substitute for meat in sandwiches, tacos, and burritos; in veggie-loaves and veggie-patties
Vegetarian gravy	Loma Linda's Low Fat All Vegetable Gravy Quik (Onion and Country Style) Gravy Mix and Fat Free Vegetarian Chicken Style Gravy Mix	On meat analogs, potatoes, etc.
Veggie-dogs (canned)	Countrylife's Country Frank; Loma Linda's Big Franks and Low Fat Big Franks	In sandwiches; on the grill
Veggie-dogs (frozen)	Nature Touch; Veggie Cuisine's (YVES) Jumbo Veggie Dog; New Menu; Lightlife Tofu Pups	In sandwiches; on the grill
Yogurt, nondairy	Nancy's Cultured Soy; White Wave Dairyless Yogurt	As a substitute for dairy yogurts, eaten alone or used in sauces, dips, and other recipes

VEGAN DESSERTS

Being a vegan does not mean having to give up desserts. As veganism becomes more popular, dairyless and eggless dessert items are becoming available. Your other option is to make your own sweet treats.

Purchasing Vegan Desserts

There are some commercial desserts and pastries that do not contain eggs, butter, milk, or other dairy products, but they are very few—for example, some fruit pies, such as apple, berry; some cookies, especially oatmeal. Remember this rule of thumb: Before you purchase anything, read the ingredients. You might also choose to call the manufacturer to confirm that there is no eggs or dairy in the product.

If making your own desserts, there are many vegan alternatives that you can use. Vegan cream cheese, sour cream, and milks, as well as a few dairyless ice creams, are listed in Table 20.5, page 228. Table 20.6, below, offers additional ideas. Most of these products can be found in your local health food store.

Preparing Vegan Desserts

I never substitute products for the eggs, milk, and other dairy products when I bake. I simply eliminate them from the recipe, and all of my desserts come out just as delicious. Most people cannot even tell that the desserts contain no animal products. But if you would like to make substitutions, Table 20.6 provides several options. Note that silken tofu is an excellent substitute that can be used to make puddings, custards, and fillings in desserts like banana cream pie.

Storing Vegan Desserts

Apply the same storage rules to desserts as you would to bread products. The desserts should be eaten within a few weeks of when they were made.

Table 20.6. Alternative Baking Products	
Nonvegan Item	**Vegan Alternative**
Eggs	Additional water; non-dairy creamer
Cream	Non-dairy creamer; silken tofu
Milk	Nut milk; soymilk; non-dairy creamer
Butter/lard	Margarine; oil; vegetable shortening

Keep them in airtight bags or containers, and refrigerate or freeze them, especially if they contain soft fillings.

SPICES AND HERBS

If you never really seasoned your food before, it is a good idea to learn how to season foods now. Herbs are the best way to season most foods. There are many herbs from which to choose. Some favorites are:

• allspice	• cloves	• oregano
• anise	• cumin	• rosemary
• basil	• curry	• saffron
• bay leaves	• garlic powder	• sage
• caraway seeds	• ginger	• savory
• cardamom	• mace	• tarragon
• cayenne pepper	• marjoram	• thyme
• chili powder	• nutmeg	• turmeric
• cinnamon	• onion powder	

Other seasonings that I frequently use and that replace chicken- or beef-based seasonings are: *Top Ramen Oriental Seasoning; El Paso/Ortega Taco Seasoning; Washington Seasoning and Broth* (golden; rich brown; onion; vegetable); *La Choy* and *Kikoman's* soy sauce; various brands of salsa; *Vegit All Purpose Seasoning; Organic Country Vegetable Harvest Bouillon Cubes;* and *Worthington's Savonex Flavoring* concentrate. In addition, when making spaghetti sauce, beans, scrambled tofu, vegetables, homemade tacos, veggie-burgers, vegan meatloaf, and fried rice, I dice one or more of the following and add them to the recipe: canned olives; cilantro; fresh celery; fresh garlic; fresh onions; fresh/canned mushrooms; and green/red/yellow bell peppers; and parsley.

Hopefully, this chapter—and this book—will assist you in making the transition to veganism. To be a successful vegan does not simply mean avoiding meat, eggs, and dairy foods; it means learning to prepare healthful and delicious meals, and it means taking an active role in improving your life and your world.

Appendix A

Nutrient Intakes, Food Tables, and Portion Information

This appendix contains a number of tables providing basic nutrient and food information. Table A.1 lists general requirements, while Tables A.2 through A.11 help you identify vegetarian foods that are rich in specific nutrients and other healthful components (such as fiber). Also, Table A.12 lists healthy portion sizes. Please note that all of the foods included in the following tables are vegan food items. Unless otherwise stated, the information is adapted from J. Pennington's *Bowes and Church's Food Values of Portions Commonly Used* (Sixteenth Edition); Whitney, Cataldo, and Rolfes's "The Table of Food Competition," from *Understanding Normal and Clinical Nutrition;* and/or my own label reading.

Table A.1. Nutrient Intakes

Vitamin/ Mineral	Best Vegetarian Sources	DRI	Probable Optimal intakes
Vitamin A/ Beta carotene	Green and yellow fruits and vegetables	5,000 IU*	5,000–10,000 IU
Vitamin B$_1$ (thiamin)	Whole grain and enriched grain products	1.0–1.5 mg	1.2–50 mg
Vitamin B$_2$ (riboflavin)	Milk and dairy foods, enriched bread and grain products, green leafy vegetables, nuts	1.0–1.6 mg	1.3–50 mg
Vitamin B$_3$ (niacin)	Peanut butter, legumes, enriched and fortified grain products	14–18 mg	15–35 mg
Vitamin B$_5$ (pantothenic acid)	Whole grain cereals, legumes	5–7 mg	5–20 mg
Vitamin B$_6$ (pyridoxine)	Whole grains, legumes, nuts	1.2–2.0 mg	1.5–50 mg
Vitamin B$_{12}$ (cobalamin)	Fortified cereal and plant milks, eggs, milk, and other dairy products	2.4–2.8 mcg	2.4–10 mcg
Vitamin C	Fruits and vegetables, especially citrus fruits	60 mg	150–1,000 mg
Vitamin D	Vitamin D-fortified soy or dairy foods, eggs, sunlight	5–15 mcg or 200–600 IU	10–15 mcg or 400–600 IU
Vitamin E	Vegetable oils, nuts, seeds, wheat germ, leafy green vegetables	30 IU	200–400 IU
Vitamin K	Leafy green vegetables	None determined	65–80 mcg
Biotin	Eggs, yeast breads, cereals	30–35 mcg	300 mcg
Boron	Fruits, vegetables	None determined	3–6 mg
Calcium	Milk and dairy foods, dark green leafy vegetables, calcium-set tofu, calcium-fortified soymilk and orange juice	1,000– 1,300 mg	1,200– 1,500 mg (for vegans: 800–1,500 mg)

Table A.1. Nutrient Intakes (cont.)

Vitamin/ Mineral	Best Vegetarian Sources	DRI	Probable Optimal intakes
Choline	Egg yolk, whole grains	425–550 mg	375–550 mg
Chromium	Eggs, whole grain products	120 mcg*	50–200 mcg
Copper	Nuts, seeds	2 mg	2–3 mg
Fluoride	Tea made with fluoridated water	2.9–3.1 mg	3.0–5.0 mg
Folate	Leafy vegetables, legumes, fruits, wheat germ, fortified cereal	400–600 mcg	400–800 mcg
Iodine	Salt, foods grown in iodine-rich soil	150 mcg*	150–200 mcg
Iron	Legumes, whole grains, nuts, fortified cereal	18 mg*	15–30 mg
Magnesium	Legumes, nuts, whole grains	310–400 mg	500–1,000 mg
Manganese	Nuts, seeds, whole grains	2 mg	2–15 mg
Molybdenum	Milk, legumes, bread, grain products	75 mcg*	75–250 mcg
Phosphorus	Eggs, milk, legumes, nuts	700–1,250 mg	1,200–1,500 mg
Potassium	Fruits, vegetables	3,500 mg**	4,000 mg
Selenium	Grain products and seeds grown in selenium-rich soil	70 mcg*	100 mcg
Sodium	Salt, processed foods	2,400 mg**	2,000–3,000 mg
Zinc	Eggs, milk, whole grains, wheat germ, miso	15 mg*	15–25 mg

*DRI not available; RDI given

**DRI not available; DV given

References: *The Real Vitamin and Mineral Book* by Shari Lieberman, PhD, and Nancy Bruning; *Vitamins, Herbs, Minerals & Supplements: The Complete Guide* by Dr. Griffith; *The American Dietetic Association's Complete Food & Nutrition Guide* by R.K. Duyff.

Table A.2. Calcium-Rich Foods

Cooked Vegetables and Vegetable Juice

Food	Calcium (mg)	Food	Calcium (mg)
Acorn squash, baked (1 cup)	90	Kale,* frozen (1 cup)	180
Beet greens, drained (1 cup)	164	Kale,* raw (1 cup)	94
Bok choy, drained (1 cup)	158	Mustard greens,* frozen (1 cup)	150
Broccoli,* frozen (1 cup)	94	Mustard greens,* raw (1 cup)	104
Butternut squash, baked (1 cup)	100	Okra, frozen (1 cup)	176
Chinese pak-choi cabbage* (1 cup)	158	Oriental radish, dried (½ cup)	365
Collard greens, frozen (1 cup)	358	Turnip greens,* canned (1 cup)	276
Dandelion greens, chopped (1 cup)	146	Turnip greens,* frozen (1 cup)	250

Fruits

Food	Calcium (mg)	Food	Calcium (mg)
Cherimoya, raw (1 medium)	126	Orange juice, calcium-fortified (1 cup)	200–240
Dates, chopped (1 cup)	58	Roselle, raw (1 cup)	123
Figs, dried (10)	269		

Grains

Food	Calcium (mg)	Food	Calcium (mg)
Amarenth (1 cup)	298	Soy meal, defatted (1 cup)	297
Corn meal with wheat flour added (1 cup)	508	Soybean flour, defatted (1 cup)	241
Corn tortilla (2)	84	Soybean flour, low-fat (1 cup)	165
Quinoa (1 cup)	102	Wheat flour, self-rising (1 cup)	422

* A food from which calcium is absorbed well by the body.

Table A.2. Calcium-Rich Foods (cont.)

Legumes/Soy products

Food	Calcium (mg)	Food	Calcium (mg)
Agar seaweed, dried (1 oz)	179	Soybeans* (1 cup)	175
Black-eye peas, immature (1 cup)	212	Soymage* cheese (1 cup)	200
California kidney beans (1 cup)	116	Soymilk (1 cup)	200–400
French beans (1 cup)	111	Tempeh (1 cup)	154
Great Northern beans (1 cup)	121	Tofu, calcium-set* (1/2 cup)	260–516
Hummus (1 cup)	124	White beans (1 cup)	161
Miso (1/2 cup)	92	White Wave Dairyless Yogurt* (6 oz)	200–280
Natto (1/2 cup)	191	Winged beans (1 cup)	244
Navy beans (1 cup)	128	Yellow beans (1 cup)	110
Soy nuts (1/2 cup)	232		

Nuts/Seeds

Food	Calcium (mg)	Food	Calcium (mg)
Almond meal (1 oz)	120	Cottonseed meal (1 oz)	143
Almonds (1 oz)	70–100		

Miscellaneous

Food	Calcium (mg)	Food	Calcium (mg)
Basil, ground (1 tbsp)	90	Rice milk, calcium-fortified (1 cup)	200–300
Blackstrap molasses (2 tbsp)	344	Soy sauce (2 tbsp)	89
Calumet baking powder (1 tsp)	241	Tortula yeast (1 oz)	120
Carob flour (1 cup)	359		

* A food from which calcium is absorbed well by the body.

Table A.3. Fiber-Rich Foods

Fruits

Food	Fiber (g)	Food	Fiber (g)
Apple (1 cup)	3.0–5.0	Prunes, dried (10)	6.0
Apples, dried (10)	8.0	Raisins ($\frac{1}{2}$ cup)	3.5
Blackberries or blueberries (1 cup)	10.0	Raspberries, fresh (1 cup)	5.8–8.0
Dates, dried (10)	4.2	Sapodilla, raw (1 medium)	9.0
Figs (10)	7.0–21.0	Strawberries, raw (1 cup)	3.9
Pear (1 medium)	4.0–6.0		
Pear halves, dried (10)	10.7–19.0		

Grains (see also, Cereals)

Food	Fiber (g)	Food	Fiber (g)
Barley, pearled (1 cup)	4.0	Wheat bran ($\frac{1}{2}$ cup)	12.7
Brown rice (1 cup)	3.3	Wheat germ ($\frac{1}{4}$ cup)	4.4
Oatmeal (1 cup)	4.0	Whole wheat bread (2 slices)	3.2

Legumes/Soy Products

Food	Fiber (g)	Food	Fiber (g)
Black beans (1 cup)	15.0	Lima beans (1 cup)	13.5–18.0
Black-eye peas (1 cup)	21.0	Lima beans, baby (1 cup)	7.8
Chickpeas (1 cup)	11.0	Miso ($\frac{1}{2}$ cup)	7.5
Hummus (1 cup)	4.0	Navy beans (1 cup)	6.6
Kidney beans (1 cup)	19.0	Pink beans (1 cup)	7.4
Lentils (1 cup)	7.9		

Nuts/Seeds

Food	Fiber (g)	Food	Fiber (g)
Almonds (1 oz)	2.0–3.5	Pistachios (1 oz)	3.0
Mixed nuts (1 oz)	2.5		

Table A.3. Fiber-Rich Foods (cont.)

Cereals

Food	Fiber (g)	Food	Fiber (g)
Cream of Rye, cooked ($\frac{2}{3}$ cup)	5.4	Kellogg's *Mini Wheats* ($\frac{3}{4}$ cup)	5.0
Kellogg's *All Bran* ($\frac{1}{3}$ cup)	10.0	General Mills' *Raisin Bran* (1 cup)	4.0
Kellogg's *Bran Flakes* ($\frac{3}{4}$ cup)	5.0	Oat bran, cooked ($\frac{1}{2}$ cup)	4.2
Kellogg's *Bran Buds* ($\frac{1}{3}$ cup)	8.0		

Miscellaneous

Food	Fiber (g)	Food	Fiber (g)
Brewer's yeast (1 tbsp)	3	Sesame seeds ($\frac{1}{4}$ cup)	6

Table A.4. Folate-Rich Foods

Legumes/Soy Products

Food	Folate (mg)	Food	Folate (mg)
Baked beans (1 cup)	60–122	Lentils, boiled (1 cup)	358
Black beans, boiled (1 cup)	256	Lima beans, baby, boiled (1 cup)	273
Black-eye peas, immature (1 cup)	209	Mingo beans (1 cup)	170
Black turtle beans (1 cup)	158	Mung beans (1 cup)	321
Bread beans (1 cup)	177	Navy beans (1 cup)	255
Chickpeas, boiled (1 cup)	282	Pinto beans, boiled (1 cup)	294
Cowpeas (1 cup)	242		
Cranberry beans, boiled (1 cup)	366	Soybean nuts ($\frac{1}{2}$ cup)	176
Great Northern beans, boiled (1 cup)	181	Split peas, boiled (1 cup)	130
Hummus (1 cup)	146	Winged beans (1 cup)	245
Kidney beans (1 cup)	229	Yard-long beans (1 cup)	249

Table A.4. Folate-Rich Foods (cont.)
Fruits and Vegetables

Food	Folate (mg)	Food	Folate (mg)
Asparagus ($\frac{1}{2}$ cup)	132	Brussels sprouts (1 cup)	94
Avocado (1 medium)	113–162	Okra, frozen ($\frac{1}{2}$ cup)	134
Beets, sliced, boiled, drained (1 cup)	90	Orange juice, from concentrate (1 cup)	109
Broccoli, fresh, boiled (1 cup)	90	Spinach ($\frac{1}{2}$ cup)	131

Table A.5. Iron-Rich Foods
Legumes/Soy Products

Food	Iron (mg)	Food	Iron (mg)
Adzuki beans (1 cup)	4.60	Lentils (1 cup)	6.59
Black beans (1 cup)	3.60	Lima beans, baby (1 cup)	4.50
Black turtle beans (1 cup)	5.27	Mingo beans (1 cup)	3.14
Black-eye peas (1 cup)	4.30	Moth beans (1 cup)	5.56
Broad beans (1 cup)	2.54	Miso ($\frac{1}{2}$ cup)	3.78
Cowpeas (1 cup)	5.22	Natto ($\frac{1}{2}$ cup)	7.57
Cranberry beans (1 cup)	3.70	Navy beans (1 cup)	4.50
Garbonzo beans/ chickpeas (1 cup)	4.74	Pinto beans (1 cup)	4.47
		Pink beans (1 cup)	3.89
Great Northern beans (1 cup)	3.77	Soy nuts (1 oz)	1.26
		Soybeans (1 cup)	8.84
Hummus (1 cup)	3.87	Tofu (1 cup)	6.65
Kidney beans (1 cup)	5.20		

Nuts/Seeds

Food	Iron (mg)	Food	Iron (mg)
Almonds (1 oz)	1.38	Pistachios (1 oz)	1.92
Cashews (1 oz)	1.70	Pumpkin seeds (1 oz)	4.25
Cottonseed flour (1 oz)	3.57	Sesame seeds (1 oz)	4.19
Mixed nuts (1 oz)	1.05	Sunflower seeds (1 oz)	1.98
Peanuts (1 oz)	1.18		

Table A.5. Iron-Rich Foods (cont.)

Fruits

Food	Iron (mg)	Food	Iron (mg)
Apricots, dried/cooked (10 halves)	1.65	Mulberries, raw (1 cup)	2.59
Banana, dried slices (1 cup)	1.15	Peaches, dried (10)	5.28
Cherries, sour, pitted (1 cup)	3.34	Pears, dried (10 halves)	3.68
Cherimoya (1 medium)	2.74	Prune juice, canned (1 cup)	3.03
Dates, chopped (1 cup)	2.14	Prunes, dried (10)	2.08
Figs, dried (10)	4.18	Raisins (½ cup)	1.30
Longans, dried (3.5 oz)	5.40	Tamarind, raw (1 cup)	3.36

Vegetables

Food	Iron (mg)	Food	Iron (mg)
Agar seaweed (1 oz)	6.00	Spinach, from raw (1 cup)	6.42
Artichokes, Jerusalem (1 cup)	5.10	Spirulina (1 ounce)	8.08
Potato, baked, skin on (1)	2.75	Swiss chard (½ cup)	1.99
Pumpkin, canned (1 cup)	3.40	Tomato paste (¼ cup)	1.96

Miscellaneous

Food	Iron (mg)	Food	Iron (mg)
Blackstrap molasses (2 tbsp)	7.00	Dill weed (1 tbsp)	1.50
Brewer's yeast (1 oz)	4.90	Tortula yeast (1 oz)	5.50
		Carob flour (1 cup)	3.03
Coconut milk (1 cup)	7.46	Wheat germ, toasted (¼ cup)	2.58

Be sure to consume fruits and vegetables rich in vitamin C with your meals, in order to increase your iron absorption.

Table A.6. Isoflavone Content in Selected Soyfoods

Soyfood	Isoflavone Content (mg)	Soyfood	Isoflavone Content (mg)
Miso ($\frac{1}{2}$ cup)	40	Tempeh ($\frac{1}{2}$ cup)	40
Soy flour ($\frac{1}{2}$ cup)	50	Textured soy protein, cooked ($\frac{1}{2}$ cup)	35
Soybeans, cooked ($\frac{1}{2}$ cup)	35		
Soymilk ($\frac{1}{2}$ cup)	40	Tofu ($\frac{1}{2}$ cup)	40
Soynuts (1 oz)	40	*White Wave Silk Dairyless Yogurt (6 oz)*	30

From U.S. 1998 Soyfoods Directory

Table A.7. Protein-Rich Foods

Grains/Starches

Food	Protein (g)	Food	Protein (g)
Barley (1 cup)	5.0	Wheat germ, toasted ($\frac{1}{4}$ cup)	8.0
Brown rice (1 cup)	5.0		
Couscous (1 cup)	6.8	Whole grain breads (2 slices/1 bagel)	8.0–10.0
Pasta, regular/ whole wheat (1 cup)	7.0–8.0	Whole grain cereal, cold (see box)	5.0–9.0

Legumes/Soy Products

Food	Protein (g)	Food	Protein (g)
Legumes/beans (1 cup)	12.0–16.0	Tempeh ($\frac{1}{2}$ cup/4 oz)	16.0–19.0
Seitan ($\frac{1}{2}$ cup)	24.0	Tofu, firm ($\frac{1}{2}$ cup/4 oz)	8.0–20.0
Soymilks/soy beverages (8 oz/1 cup)	4.0–10.0		

Miscellaneous

Food	Protein (g)	Food	Protein (g)
Nuts/nutbutters (1 oz)	4.0–7.0	Vegetarian meat analogs (see container/ package)	10.0–18.0

Table A.8. Vitamin B₁₂-Fortified Foods

Product	Vitamin B₁₂ (mcg)	Product	Vitamin B₁₂ (mcg)
Countrylife's *Tender Chops* (see package)	7.3	*Red Star T-6635 Yeast*, mini flakes (1½ tsp)	2.0
EdenSoy Extra soymilk (8 oz)	4.0	*Red Star T-6635 Yeast*, large flakes (2 tsp)	2.0
General Mills' *Total Whole Grain* (¾ cup)	2.0	Soymilk/soy beverages (see label)	1.5–3.0
Kellogg's *Product 19* (1 cup)	2.0	Worthington's *Tuno,* canned (see label)	1.8
Loma Linda's Lowfat Big Franks, canned (see label)	1.2	*YVES Canadian Veggie Bacon* (see package)	1.2

Note: Vegetable and legume sources said to be rich in vitamin B₁₂, such as seaweed, tempeh, and miso, are not dependable sources. Be sure to check the label of any product that you believe to contain vitamin B₁₂.

Table A.9. Vitamin C-Rich Foods

Fruits

Food	Vitamin C (mg)	Food	Vitamin C (mg)
Acerola, raw (½ cup)	822	Lychees, raw (10 medium)	72
Cantaloupe (1 cup)	68	Orange, fresh/juice (1 fruit/1 cup)	70–124
Grapefruit, fresh/juice (1 fruit/1 cup)	60–248	Papaya (1 cup)	92
		Pommelo (1 medium)	116
Guava (1 medium)	165	Strawberries (1 cup)	85
Kiwi (1 fruit)	75		

Vegetables

Food	Vitamin C (mg)	Food	Vitamin C (mg)
Broccoli (1 cup)	116	Kohlrabi (1 cup)	88
Brussels sprouts, boiled (1 cup)	96	Mustard spinach, boiled (1 cup)	118
Cauliflower, raw (1 cup)	72	Sweet yellow bell pepper (1 large)	341
Green chili peppers, hot raw (1)	109		

Table A.10. Vitamin D-Rich Foods

Dry Cereals

Product	Vitamin D (IU)	Food	Vitamin D (IU)
General Mills' *Whole Grain Total* (¾ cup)	40	Kellogg's *Product 19* (1 cup)	40

Non-dairy Drinks

Product	Vitamin D (IU)	Food	Vitamin D (IU)
EdenSoy Extra soymilk (8 oz)	40	*West Brae Natural West Soy* non-fat soy beverage (8 oz)	100
Health Valley *Fat Free SoyMoo Non-dairy* soy drink (8 oz)	100	*West Brae Natural West Soy Plus* soy beverage (8 oz)	100
Rice Dream rice milk (8 oz)	100	*White Wave Silk Soymilk* (8 oz)	120

Table A.11. Zinc-Rich Foods

Grains

Food	Zinc (mg)	Food	Zinc (mg)
Barley, pearled cereal (1 cup)	1.29	Kellogg's *All Bran* (⅓ cup)	3.75
Buckwheat flour (1 cup)	3.75	Whole wheat bread (2 slices)	1.00
Corn meal, whole grain (1 cup)	2.21	Whole wheat flour (1 cup)	3.52

Nuts/Seeds

Food	Zinc (mg)	Food	Zinc (mg)
Brazil nuts (1 oz)	1.30	Pumpkin seeds (1 oz)	2.12
Cashew butter (1 oz)	1.47	Sesame butter (1 tbsp)	1.46
Cashews (1 oz)	1.59	Sesame kernels (1 oz)	2.90
Cottonseed meal (1 oz)	3.50	Sesame meal (1 oz)	2.91
Peanuts (1 oz)	1.86	Sunflower seeds (1 oz)	1.42
Pecans (1 oz)	1.55		

Table A.11. Zinc-Rich Foods

Legumes/Soy Products

Food	Zinc (mg)	Food	Zinc (mg)
Adzuki beans (1 cup)	4.06	Natto ($\frac{1}{2}$ cup)	2.67
Black beans (1 cup)	1.92	Navy beans (1 cup)	1.93
Black-eye peas (1 cup)	1.70	Pinto beans (1 cup)	1.85
Cowpeas/catjang (1 cup)	3.20	Soybean nuts (1 oz)	1.36
Garbonzo beans/		Soybeans (1 cup)	1.98
chickpeas (1 cup)	2.51	Split-peas (1 cup)	1.96
Hummus (1 cup)	2.70	Tofu ($\frac{1}{2}$ cup)	1.98
Kidney beans (1 cup)	1.89	White beans (1 cup)	2.46
Lentils (1 cup)	2.50	Winged beans (1 cup)	2.48
Lima beans, baby (1 cup)	1.87	Yard-long beans (1 cup)	1.84
Lupins (1 cup)	2.29	Yellow beans (1 cup)	1.87
Miso ($\frac{1}{2}$ cup)	4.50		

Miscellaneous

Food	Zinc (mg)	Food	Zinc (mg)
Wheat germ, toasted ($\frac{1}{2}$ cup)	4.73	Tortula dried yeast (1 oz)	3.60

Table A.12. Healthy Portion Sizes

Fruits

Type of Food	Serving Size	Type of Food	Serving Size
Canned	$\frac{1}{2}$ cup	Fresh	1 medium
Dried	10 pieces	Juices	$\frac{3}{4}$ cup; 6 oz

Meat Alternatives

Type of Food	Serving Size	Type of Food	Serving Size
Beans, cooked	$\frac{1}{2}$ cup	Tempeh	4 oz
Canned/frozen dried meat substitutes	on label	Tofu	4 oz

Table A.12. Healthy Portion Sizes (cont.)

Nuts

Type of Food	Serving Size	Type of Food	Serving Size
Nuts	1 oz	Nutbutters	1 oz

Starches

Type of Food	Serving Size	Type of Food	Serving Size
Breads	1 slice	Pasta	$\frac{1}{2}$ cup
Cold cereals	$\frac{3}{4}$ cup	Rice	$\frac{1}{2}$ cup
Hot cereals	$\frac{1}{2}$ cup	Soups	$\frac{1}{2}$ cup

Vegetables

Type of Food	Serving Size	Type of Food	Serving Size
Fresh, cooked	$\frac{1}{2}$ cup	Raw	$\frac{1}{2}$ cup
Juice	4 oz		

Appendix B

Suggested Cookbooks and Guides

There are many vegetarian and vegan cookbooks from which to choose. Below are recommendations to get you started on your collection. Please note that if there is an asterisk (*) after the title, the cookbook is specifically vegan. *A Celebration of Wellness: An Easy to Use Vegetarian Cookbook . . . With Over 300 Lowfat and Nonfat Heart Healthy, No Dairy, No Cholesterol Recipes* by James Levin and Natalie Cederquest (Garden City Park, NY: Avery Publishing Group, 1995).

Cooking With the Right Side of the Brain: Creative Vegetarian Cooking by Vicki Rae Chelf and Vicky Hudon (Garden City Park, NY: Avery Publishing Group, 1990).

Follow Your Heart's Vegetarian Soup Cookbook by Janice Cook Migliaccio (Santa Barbara, CA: Woodbridge Press Publishing Company, 1983).

Foods From Mother Earth by Maura D. Shaw and Sydna Altschuler Byrne (Shawangunk Press, 1994).

Foods That Heal by Bernard Jensen (Garden City Park, NY: Avery Publishing Group, 1993).

The Garden of Earthly Delights Cookbook: Gourmet Vegetarian Cooking by Shea MacKenzie (Garden City Park, NY: Avery Publishing Group, 1995).

The Harvest Collection: A Vegetarian Cookbook for All Seasons by Gardner Merchant (Garden City Park, NY: Avery Publishing Group, 1994).

The High Road to Health: A Vegetarian Cookbook by Lindsay Wagner and Ariane Spade (St. Louis, MO: Fireside Books, 1994).

The Joy of Juicing Recipe Guide: Creative Cooking With Your Juicer by Gary Null and Shelly Null (Garden City Park, NY: Avery Publishing Group, 1992).

Lean and Luscious and Meatless by Bobbie Hinman and Millie Snyder (Rocklin, CA: Prima Publishing, 1998).

The Meatless Gourmet: Easy Lowfat Favorites by Bobbie Hinman (Rocklin, CA: Prima Publishing, 1996).

The New Farm Vegetarian Cookbook by Louise Hagler and Dorothy Bates (Summertown, TN: Book Publishing Company, 1989).

The New Laurel's Kitchen: A Handbook for Vegetarian Cooking and Nutrition by Laurel Robertson, Carol Flinders, and Brian Ruppenthal (Berkeley, CA: Ten Speed Press, 1986).

The Sensuous Vegetarian Barbecue: A Hot and Healthful Collection of Recipes, Marinades, and Grilling Tips by Vicki Rae Chelf and Dominique Biscotti (Garden City Park, NY: Avery Publishing Group, 1994).

Simply Vegan: Quick Vegetarian Meals* by Debra Wasserman, PhD, nutrition section by Reed Mangels (Baltimore, MD: Vegetarian Resource Group, 1999).

The Tofu Book: The New American Cuisine* by John Paino and Lisa Messinger (Garden City Park, NY: Avery Publishing Group, 1991).

Vegan Delights: Gourmet Vegetarian Specialties* by John Robbins and Jeanne Marie Martin (Madeira Park, BC: Harbour Publishing Company, 1997).

The Vegan Gourmet: Full Flavor and Variety With Over 100 Delicious Recipes* by Susann Geiskopt-Hadler and Mindy Toomay (Rocklin, CA: Prima Publishing, 1999).

Vegan Vittles: Recipes Inspired by the Critters of Farm Sanctuary* by Joanne Stepaniak and Suzanne Havala (Summerton, TN: Book Publishing Company, 1996).

Vegetarian Christmas: Festive Feasts for All the Family by Rose Elliot (Thorsons Publishing, 1995).

Vegetarian Cooking for People With Diabetes by Patricia Leshane and Patricia Mozzer (Summerton, TN: Book Publishing Company, 1994).

Vegetarian Times Complete Cookbook by the editors of *Vegetarian Times* and Lucy Moll (New York, NY: Macmillan General Reference, 1995).

Some cookbooks are not necessarily vegetarian but still can be of great use in coming up with meal ideas, especially the ones that include large photographs of prepared dishes. Often, cookbooks that concentrate on a specific type of food, such as pasta, vegetables, or breads, contain beautiful pictures that will spark your creativity. They offer added help in finding new ways to prepare staple products in your diet. I suggest the following books:

Breads

The Laurel's Kitchen Bread Book: A Guide to Whole-Grain Bread-Making by Laurel Robertson, with Carol Flinders and Bronwen Godfrey (New York: Random House, 1985).

Pasta, Starches

The Essential Pasta Cookbook (Portland, OR: Whitecap Books, 1998).

The Pasta Gourmet: Creative Pasta Recipes from Appetizers to Desserts by Sunny Baker and Michelle Sbraga (Garden City Park, NY: Avery Publishing Group, 1995).

Fruits and Vegetables

Fresh From the Farmer's Market: Year-Round Recipes for the Pick of the Crop by Janet Kessel Fletcher, photographs by Vectoria Pearson, and introduction by Alice Waters (San Francisco, CA: Chronicle Books, 1997).

Vegetables on the Side: The Complete Guide to Buying and Cooking by Sallie Y. Williams (New York, NY: Macmillan General Reference, 1998).

Victory Garden Cookbook by Marion Morash (New York, NY: Random House, Inc., 1982).

Legumes

Boutique Bean Pot by Kathleen Mayes and Sandra Gottfried (Batavia, IL: Woodbridge Press Publishing, 1992).

Bean Cuisine by Janet Horsley (Garden City Park, NY: Avery Publishing Group, 1983).

Nuts and Seeds

Not Milk . . . Nut Milks: 40 of the Most Original Dairy-Free Recipes Ever by Candia Lea Cole (Batavia, IL: Woodbridge Press Publishing, 1997).

Many helpful books are available to vegetarians/vegans today. You can easily find informative guides that will provide you with more information; simply visit your library or bookstore, or do a search on the World Wide Web. Below, I have listed a few books that come highly recommended.

Diet for a Small Planet (20th Anniversary Edition) by Frances Moore Lappé (New York, NY: Ballantine Books, 1992).

Diet for a New America: How Your Food Choices Affect Your Health, Happiness and the Future of Life on Earth by John Robbins (Tiburon, CA: HJ Kramer, Inc., 1987).

Pregnancy, Children and the Vegan Diet by Michael Klaper (Gentle World, 1988).

Vegan Nutrition: Pure and Simple by Michael Klaper (Gentle World, 1987).

A Vegetarian Sourcebook: The Nutrition, Ecology, and Ethics of a Natural Foods Diet by Keith Akers (Baltimore, MD: Vegetarian Resource Group, 1993).

Appendix C

Resource Directory

B elow are listed a number of helpful sources. They will provide you with further information on issues of vegetarianism, nutrition, and/or health.

Vegetarian Magazines

U.S. Soyfoods Directory
Indiana Soybean Board
423 West South Street
Lebanon, IN 46052–2461
Phone: (800) TALKSOY
E-mail: info@soyfoods.com

Vegetarian Journal
The Vegetarian Resource Group
PO Box 1463
Baltimore, MD 21203
Phone: (410) 366–VEGE
Subscription: 1 year at $20.00;
bimonthly publication

Vegetarian Times
4 High Ridge Park
Stamford, CT 06905

Subscription phone:
(800)–829–3340
Subscription: 12 issues for $19.95;
24 issues for $29.95
General phone: (203) 322–2900
Editorial questions:
(203) 321–1796
Fax: (203) 322–1966
Website:
   http://www.vegetariantimes.com

Vegetarian Voice
North American Vegetarian Society
PO Box 72
Dolgeville, NY 13329
Phone: (518) 568–7970
Magazine published quarterly.

Vegetarian Organizations

American Vegan Society
PO Box H
Malaga, NJ 08328
Phone: (609) 694–2887
Membership: $18.00 per year

North American Vegetarian Society
PO Box 72
Dolgeville, NY 13329
Phone: (518) 568–7970
Membership: $20.00 per year
Website: http://www.cyberveg.org/
  navs

Physicians Committee for
Responsible Medicine (PCRM)
5100 Wesconsin Avenue, Suite 404
Washington, D.C. 20016
Phone: (202) 686–2210
Fax: (212) 686–2216
E-mail: pcrm@pcrm.org
Website: http://www.pcrm.org

Vegetarian Awareness Network
Box 321
Knoxville, TN 37901

Vegetarian Resource Group
PO Box 1463
Baltimore, MD 21203
Phone: (410) 366–VEGE
Website: http://www.vrg.org
Membership: $20.00; includes
1-year subscription to *Vegetarian
Journal*

The Vegetarian Youth Network
PO Box 1141
New Paltz, NY 12561
Website: http://www.geocities.com/
  RainForest/Vines/4482
Also write to the Vegetarian Youth
Pen-Pal Directory, at the same
address.

Health Organizations

American Cancer Society (ACS)
1599 Clifton Road, N.E.
Atlanta, GA 30329
Phone: (800) ACS–2345 or
(404) 320–3333
Website: http://www.cancer.org

American Diabetes Association
1660 Duke Street
Alexandria, VA 22314–0592
Phone: (800) 232–3472 or
(703) 549–1500
Website: http://www.diabetes.org

American Dietetic Association
216 West Jackson Boulevard,
Suite 800
Chicago, IL 60606–6995
Phone: (800) 366–1655
Website: http://www.eatright.org

American Heart Association
7272 Greenville Avenue
Dallas, TX 75231
Phone: (800) AHA–USA1
Website:
  http://www.americanheart.org

American Medical Association
(AMA)
515 North State Street
Chicago, IL 60610
Phone: (312) 464–5000
Website: http://www.ama-assn.org

American Menopause
Foundation, Inc.
350 Fifth Avenue, Suite 2822
New York, NY 10118
Phone: (212) 714–2398

Arthritis Foundation
(National Office)
1314 Spring Street, N.W.
Atlanta, GA 30309
Phone: (800) 283–7800 or
(404) 872–7100

National Cancer Institute
Cancer Information Service (CIS)
National Institutes of Health
Building 31, Room 10A24
9000 Rockville Pike
Bethesda, MD 20892
Phone: (800) 422–6237
Website: http://www.nci.nih.gov

National Eating Disorders
Organization (NEDO)
6655 South Yale
Tulsa, OK 74136
Phone: (918) 481–4044
Website: http://www.laureate.com

National Health Information Center
PO Box 1133
Washington, DC 20013–1133
Phone: (800) 336–4797 or
(301) 565–4167
Website: http://nhic-nt.health.org

National Institute of Diabetes and
Digestive and Kidney Diseases
(NIDDK)
National Institutes of Health
Building 31, Room 9A04
31 Center Drive MSC 2560
Bethesda, MD 20892–2560
Phone: (301) 496–3583
Website: http://www.niddk.nih.gov

National Kidney Foundation
30 East 33rd Street, Suite 1100
New York, NY 10016
Phone: (800) 622–9010
Website: http://www.kidney.org

National Osteoporosis Foundation
2100 M Street, NW, Suite 602
Washington, DC 20037
Phone: (800) 223–9994

PMS Access
Women's Health America Group
PO Box 9362
Madison, WI 53715
Phone: (800) 222–4767 or
(608) 833–4767

Additional Helpful Websites

EnviroLink: The Online
Environmental Community
http://www.envirolink.org:80/
  arra/ADA.html

FARM: Farm Animal Reform
Movement
http://www.farmusa.org/

U.S. Food and Drug
Administration, "More People
Trying Vegetarian Diets," by Dixie
Farley
http://www.fda.gov/fdac/
  features/895_vegdiet.html

Vegetarian Pages
http://www.veg.org/veg/

Veggies Anonymous
http://www.geocities.com/
  HotSprings/4664/

Appendix D

Personal Fluid Intake and Food Pattern Charts

To help you keep better track of the liquids and foods that you consume daily, this appendix provides two charts. The first chart helps you record fluid intake. Aim to drink six to eight 8-ounce glasses of fluid daily. Photocopy the chart (make a copy for each week of the month) and stick it to your refrigerator door. Every time you drink a glass of water or juice, put a checkmark in the appropriate box.

The second chart offers the general daily food pattern for vegan females aged 25 to 50 years. It includes a final blank column for you to fill in your own goals. Use this table as a reference, so that you plan your meals, with the appropriate number of servings in mind.

Daily Fluid Intake Record								
	1	2	3	4	5	6	7	8
Sunday								
Monday								
Tuesday								
Wednesday								
Thursday								
Friday								
Saturday								

Personal Food Pattern Goals

Food Group	Serving Size	Suggested Servings/Day	My Serving-Number Goal
Whole grain products (bread; cereal; rice; pasta)	1 slice; ½ bagel; ½ cup	6–11	☐
Fruits; fruit juices	1 medium piece; ½ cup chopped; ½ cup dried; 6 oz	2–5	☐
Vegetables; vegetable juices	½ cup cooked; 1 cup raw; 4 oz	2–4	☐
Dark green, leafy vegetables		1–3	☐
Tofu; meat analogs; soymilk/ soy beverages; other protein-rich soy products	4 oz	2–4	☐
Legumes/beans	½ cup	1–3	☐
Nuts and seeds (including nutbutters)	1 oz; 2 tbsp	1–2	☐
Vitamin B_{12}- and vitamin D-fortified foods (for example, soymilk; dry cereals)	As specified for the food group.	1–2	☐

References

"A King Among Men," *The Vegetarian Times* (Oct, 1995): 128.

Abdulla, M, et al. "Nutrient intake and health status of vegans. Chemical analyses of diets using the duplicate portion sampling technique," *American Journal of Clinical Nutrition* 34(11) 1981: 2464–2477.

Abelow, BJ, TR Holford, and KL Insogna. "Cross-cultural association between dietary animal protein and hip fracture: a hypothesis," *Calcified Tissue International* 50(1) (1992): 14–18.

Abraham, R, et al. "Diets of Asian pregnant women in Harrow: iron and vitamins," *Human Nutrition—Applied Nutrition* 41(3) (1987): 164–173.

ADA Reports. "Position of the American Dietetic Association: Nutrition, aging, and the continuum of care," *Journal of the American Dietetic Association* 96(10) (1996): 1048–1052.

ADA Reports. "Position of the American Dietetic Association: Nutrition care for pregnant adolescents," *Journal of the American Dietetic Association* 94(4) (1994): 449–450.

ADA Reports. "Position of the American Dietetic Association: Promotion of breastfeeding," *Journal of the American Dietetic Association* 97(6) (1997): 662–666.

ADA Reports. "Position of the American Dietetic Association: Vegetarian Diets," *Journal of the American Dietetic Association* 93(11) (1993): 1317–1319.

ADA Reports. "Position of the American Dietetic Association: Vitamin and mineral supplementation," *Journal of the American Dietetic Association* 96(1) 1996: 73–77.

ADA Reports. "Position of the American Dietetic Association and the Canadian Dietetic Association: Women's health and nutrition," *Journal of the American Dietetic Association* 95(3) (1995): 362–367.

ADA Reports. "Position paper on the vegetarian approach to eating," *Journal of the American Dietetic Association* 77 (1980): 61–69.

Akesson, B, and PA Ockerman. "Selenium status in vegans and lactovegetarians," *British Journal of Nutrition* 53(2) (1985): 199–205.

Aldercreutz, CH, et al. "Soybean phytoestrogen intake and cancer risk," *Journal of Nutrition* 125(suppl 3) (1995): 737s–770s.

Aldridge, T, and H Schluback. "Water Requirements for Food Production," *Soil and Water* 38 (Fall, 1978), University of California cooperative extension, 13017; information from Paul Ehrlich and Anne Ehrlich's *Population, Resources, Environment* (San Francisco, CA: Freemna, 1972: 13–17; 75–76).

Alexander D, MJ Ball, and J Mann. "Nutrient intake and haematological status of vegetarians and age-sex matched omnivores," *European Journal of Clinical Nutrition* 48(8) (1994): 538–546.

Alexander, JW. "Specific Nutrients and the Immune Response," *Nutrition* II (suppl 2) (1995): 229–232.

Allen, R, and A Long. "Dietary sources of vitamin B_{12} for vegans and other special groups," *Journal of the Royal College of General Practitioners* 38(308) (1988): 123.

Allingr, UR, et al. "Shift from a mixed to a lactovegetarian diet: Influence on acidic lipids in fecal water—a potential risk factor for colon cancer," *American Journal of Clinical Nutrition* 50(5) (1989): 992–996.

Almendingen, K, K Trygg, and M Vatn. "Influence of the diet on cell proliferation in the large bowel and the rectum. Does a strict vegetarian diet recude the risk of intestinal cancer?", *Tidsskr Nor Laegeforen* 115(18, abstract) (1995): 2252–2256.

Alonso-Amelot, ME, et al. *Nature* 382 (1996): 587.

American Dairy Association & Dairy Council Mid East. *The Nutrition Edition* (vol 4, no 2) (1998).

American Dairy Association & Dairy Council Mid East. *The Nutrition Edition* 4(2) (1998).

American Dairy Association & Dairy Council Mid East. "Report Highlights Dietary Requirements for Calcium and Related Nutrients," *The Nutrition Edition* 3(3) (1997): 1–2.

American Diabetes Association. "Diabetes Dispatch: Seventh Annual American Diabetes Alert," *Diabetes Forecast* (Mar, 1995): 65.

"American Dietetic Association: Health implications of dietary fiber (Position Statement)," *Journal of the American Dietetic Association* 93 (1993): 1446–1447.

American Heart Association. *1997 Cardiovascular Statistics.* Dallas, TX: American Heart Association, 1998.

American Heart Association. *Heart and Stroke Facts: 1996 statistical supplement.* Dallas, TX: American Heart Association, 1997.

American Heart Association. *Heart and Stroke Facts: 1994.* Dallas, TX: American Heart Association, 1995.

American Heart Association. "High Blood Pressure Statistics," *Cardiovascular Disease Statistics,* www.americanheart.org (June 8, 1999).

American Institute for Cancer Research. "What is a plant-based diet?", *AICR Newsletter on Diet, Nutrition and Cancer* 59 (Spring, 1998): 1–3.

American Society for Bone and Mineral Research and Health Professionals' Committee for Nutrition Education. *Osteoporosis: The Silent Epidemic.* St. Louis, MO.

"An Ad We'd Like to See," *Vegetarian Times* 224 (1996): 136.

Anderson, BM, RS Gibson, and JH Sabry. "The iron and zinc status of long-term vegetarian women," *American Journal of Clinical Nutrition* 34(6) (1981): 1042–1048.

Anderson, JW, et al. "Cholesterol-lowering effects of psyllium-enriched cereal as an adjunct to a prudent diet in the treatment of mild to moderate hypercholesterolemia," *American Journal of Clinical Nutrition* 56 (1992): 93–98.

Anderson, JW, et al. "Dietary fiber and diabetics: A comprehensive review and application," *Journal of the American Dietetics Association* 87(9) (1987): 1189–1197.

Anderson, JW, BM Smith, and NJ Gustafson. "Health benefits and practical aspects of high-fiber diets," *American Journal of Clinical Nutrition* 59(suppl) (1994): 1242s–1247s.

Anthony, MS. "CHD protection by soy and its phytoestrogens: Beyond plasma lipid concentration," *Soy Connection* 3(3) (1995): 1.

Antol, Marie Nadine. *Healing Teas.* Garden City Park, NY: Avery Publishing Group, 1996.

Appel, LJ, et al. "A clinical trial of the effects of dietary patterns on blood pressure," *New England Journal of Medicine* 336 (Apr 17, 1997): 1117–1124.

Appleby, P, et al. "Emergency appendicectomy and meat consumption in the UK," *Journal of Epidemiology & Community Health* 49(6) (1995): 594–596.

Arnaud, CD, and SD Sanchez. "The role of calcium in osteoporosis," *Annual Review of Nutrition* 10 (1990): 397–414.

Arnold, C. "The Macrobiotic diet: A question of nutrition," *Oncology Nursing Forum* 11(3) (1984): 50–53.

Arntzenius, AC, et al. "Diet, lipoproteins, and the progressions of coronary atherosclerosis: The Keiden Intervention Trial," *New England Journal of Medicine* 312(13) (1985): 805–811.

Ascherio, A, et al. "Dietary iron intake and risk of coronary heart disease among men," *Circulation* 89 (1994): 969–974.

Baglieri, A, et al. "Gastro-jejunal digestion of soy-bean-milk protein in humans," *British Journal of Nutrition* 72(4) (1994): 519–532.

Bar-Sella, P, Y Rakover, and D Ratner. "Vitamin B_{12} and folate levels in long-term vegans," *Israel Journal of Medical Sciences* 26(6) (1990): 309–312.

Barbosa, JC, et al. "The relationship among adiposity, diet, and hormone concentrations in vegetarian and nonvegetarian postmenopausal women," *American Journal of Clinical Nutrition* 51(5) (1990): 798–803.

Barger-lux, RJ, and RP Heaney. "The role of calcium intake in preventing bone fragility, and certain cancers," *Journal of Nutrition* 124 (1994): 1406s–1411s.

Barnard, Neal. *Food for Life.* New York, NY: Crown Trade Paperbacks, 1993.

Barnard, ND, A Nicholson, and JL Howard. "The medical cost attributable to meat consumption," *Preventative Medicine* 24(6) (1995): 646–655.

Barnard, RJ, et al. "Long-term use of a high-complex carbohydrate, high-fiber, low-fat diet and exercise in the treatment of NIDDM patients," *Diabetes Care* 6(3) (1983): 268--273.

Beecher, C. "Cancer preventative properties of varieties of Brassica Oleracea: A review," *American Journal of Clinical Nutrition* 59 (suppl) (1994): 1166s–1170s.

Beilin, LJ. "Vegetarian and other complex diets, fats, fiber, and hypertension," *American Journal of Clinical Nutrition* 59(suppl 5) (1994): 1130s–1135s.

Beilin, LJ. "Vegetarian approach to hypertension," *Canadian Journal of Physiology and Pharmacology* 64(4) (1986): 852–855.

Beilin, LJ. "Vegetarian diets, alcohol consumption and hypertension," *Annals of the New York Academy of Sciences 676(Mar 15, 1993):* 83–91.

Beilin, LJ, et al. "Vegetarian diet and blood pressure," *Nephron* 47(suppl 1) (1987): 37–41.

Beilin, LJ, et al. "Vegetarian diets and blood pressure levels: Incidental or causal association?", *American Journal of Clinical Nutrition* 48(suppl 3) (1988): 806–810.

Beilin, LJ, and V Burke. "Vegetarian diet components, protein and blood pressure: which nutrients are important?", *Clinical & Experimental Pharmacology & Physiology* 22(3) (1995): 195–198.

Bennett, FC, and DM Ingram. "Diet and female sex hormone concentration: an intervention study for the type of fat consumed," *American Journal of Clinical Nutrition* 52(5) (1990): 808–812.

Bennion, Marion. *Introductory Foods.* New York, NY: Macmillan Publishing Company, 1990.

Benson, JE, KA Engelbert-Fenton, and PA Eisenman. "Nutritional aspects of amenorrhea in the female athlete triad," *International Journal of Sports Nutrition* 6(2) (1996): 134–135.

Bendich, A. "Biological Functions of Dietary Carotenoids," *Annals of the New York Academy of Sciences* 691(Dec 31, 1993) 61–67.

Berkow, Robert, MD, ed. in chief, Mark H. Beers, MD, assoc. ed., and Andrew J. Fletcher, MB, BChir, senior asst. ed. et al. *The Merck Manual of Medical Information, Home Edition.* Whitehouse Station, NJ: Merck & Co., Inc., 1997.

Berkow, Robert, MD, AJ Fletcher, MB, MChir, et al. *The Merck Manual of Diagnosis and*

Therapy (16th ed). Rahway, NJ: Merck Research Laboratories, 1992.

Berman, AF. "Having our soy," *Ms. Magzine* (Jan/Feb, 1996): 30–31.

Berry, EM, S Eisenberg, et al. "Effects of diets rich in monounsaturated fatty acids on plasma lipoproteins: The Jerusalem Nutrition Study. II Monounsaturated fatty acids vs. carbohydrates," *The American Journal of Clinical Nutrition* 56 (1992): 394–403.

Blumberg, JB, et al. "Better Testing for *E. Coli* Won't Guarantee Bug-Free Burgers," *Tufts University Diet & Nutrition Letter* 15(8) (1997): 3.

Blumberg, JB, et al. "Bugs in the berry patch?", *Tufts University Diet & Nutrition Letter* 14(7) (1996): 3.

Blumberg, JB, et al. "Mad Cow Disease 'Jumps' to Humans," *Tufts University Health & Nutrition Letter* 15(10) (1997): 1, 7.

Boon, T. "Teaching the immune system to fight cancer," *Scientific American* 268(30) (1993): 82–89.

Borgstrom G. "Presentation to the Annual Meeting of the American Association for the Advancement of Science" (1981) in John Robbins' *Diet for a New America*. Walpole, NH: Stillpoint, 1987: 367.

Bowman, BB, et al. "Macrobiotic diets for cancer treatment and prevention," *Journal of Clinical Oncology* 2(6) (1984): 702–711.

Brandle, E, HG Sieberth, and RE Hautmann. "Effect of chronic dietary protein intake on the renal function in healthy subjects," *European Journal of Clinical Endocrinology & Metabolism* 66(1) (1988): 140–146.

Brants, HA, et al. "Adequacy of a vegetarian diet at old age (Dutch Nutrition Surveillance System)," *Journal of the American College of Nutrition* 9(4) (1990): 292–302.

Breslau, NA, et al. "Relationship of animal protein-rich diet to kidney stone formation and calcium metabolism," *Journal of Clinical Endocrinology & Metabolism* 66(1) (1988): 140–146.

Brestrich M, J Claus, and G Blumchen. "Lactovegetarian diet: Effect on changes in body weight, lipid status, fibrinogen and lipoprotein (a) in cardiovascular patients during inpatient rehabiliation treatment," *Zeitschrift fur Kardiologie* 85(6) (1996): 418–427.

Bricklin, Mark. *The Practical Encyclopedia of Natural Healing*. New York, NY: MJF Books, 1983.

Briggs, M. "The use and misuse of vitamin supplements," *Australian Family Physician* 6(2) (1977): 145–147, 150–152.

Brockis, JG, AJ Levitt, and SM Cruthers. "The effects of vegetable and animal protein diets on calcium, urate, and oxalate excretion," *British Journal of Urology* 54(6) (1982): 590–593.

Brown, L, et al. *Vital Signs 1994*. Washington, DC: Worldwatch Institue, 1994.

Brummer, BA, and BL Drinkwater. "Nutrient intake in amenorrheic and eumenorrheic athletes," *Medical Science Sports Exercise* 19 (1987): 537.

Brune, M, L Rossander, and L Hallberg. "Iron absorption: No intestinal adaptation to a high-phytate diet," *American Journal of Clinical Nutrition* 49 (1989): 542–545.

Burr, ML, and BK Butland. "Heart disease in British vegetarians," *American Journal of Clinical Nutrition* 48(suppl 3) (1988): 830–832.

Burr, ML, and PM Sweetnam. "Vegetarianism, dietary fiber and mortality," *American Journal of Clinical Nutrition* 36(5) (1982): 873–877.

Byczkowski, JZ, and JW Fisher. "A computer program linking physiologically based pharmacokinetic model with cancer risk assessment for breast-fed infants," *Computer Methods & Programs in Biomedicine* 46(2) (1995): 155–163.

Calkings, BM, et al. "Diet, nutrition intake, and metabolism in populations at high and low risk for colon cancer," *American Journal of Clinical Nutrition* 40(suppl 4) (1984): 896–905.

Campbell, TC, and C Junski. "Diet and chronic degenerative diseases: Perspective from China," *American Journal of Clinical Nutrition* 59(suppl) (1994): 1153s–1161s.

Campbell-Brown, M, et al. "Zinc and copper in Asian pregnancies—is there evidence for a nutritional deficiency?", *British Journal of Obstetrics & Gynaecology* 92(9) (1985): 875–885.

Carter, JP, T Furman, and HR Hutcheson. "Preeclampsia and reproductive performance in a community of vegans," *Southern Medical Journal* 80(6) (1987): 692–697.

Cass, Hyla, MD. *St. John's Wort: Nature's Blues Buster.* Garden City Park, NY: Avery Publishing Group, 1998.

Cassidy, A, S Bingham, and K Setchell. "Biological effects of a diet of soy protein rich in isoflavones on the menstrual cycle of premenopausal women," *American Journal of Clinical Nutrition* 60(3) (Sep 1994): 333–340.

Chan, EL, and R Swaminathan. "The effect of high protein and high salt intake for 4 months on calcium and hydroxyproline excretion in normal and oophorectomized rats," *Journal of Laboratory & Clinical Medicine* 124(1) (1994): 37–41.

Chan, GM, et al. "Effects of increased dietary calcium intake upon the calcium and bone mineral status of lactating adolescent and adult women," *American Journal of Clinical Nutrition* 46(2) (1987): 319–323.

Chanarin, I, et al. "Megaloblastic anaemia in a vegetarian Hindu community," *Lancet* 2(8465) (1985): 1168–1172.

Chandra, RK, and S Kumari. "Nutrition and immunity: An overview," *Journal of Nutrition* 124(suppl 8) (1994): 1433s–1435s.

Chang CJ, et al. "Selenium content of Brazil nuts from two geographic locations in Brazil," *Chemosphere* 30(4) (1995): 801–802.

Chang CJ, BR Frentzel, and U Eilber. "Mortality pattern of German vegetarians after 11 years of follow-up," *Epidemiology* 3(5) (1992): 395–401.

Chiu, JF, et al. "Long-term vegetarian diet and bone mineral density in postmenopausal Taiwanese women," *Calcified Tissue International* 60(3) (1997): 245–249.

Clark, N. "Counseling the athlete with an eating disorder: a case study," *Journal of the American Dietetic Association* 94(6) (1994): 656–658.

Cleveland Clinic Foundation. *The Epidemic of the 90's: Obesity.* Willoughby Hills, OH: Cleveland Clinic Foundation.

Cleveland, LE, and AB Pfeffer. "Planning diets to meet the National Research Council's Guidelines for Reducing Cancer Risk," *Journal of the American Dietetic Association* 87 (1987): 162–168.

"Clinical Insights in Diabetes #2," adapted from AL Rosenbloom's "Emerging epidemic of type 2 diabetes in youth," *Diabetes Care* 22 (March 15, 1999): 345–354.

Cournoyer, D, and CT Caskey. "Gene therapy of the immune system," *Annual Review of Immunology* 11 (1993): 297–329.

Craig, WJ. "Iron status of vegetarians," *American Journal of Clinical Nutrition* 59(suppl) (1994): 1233s–1237s.

Craig, WJ. "Phytochemicals: New frontiers in disease prevention," *Soy Connection* 4(2) (1996): 2.

Crapo, PA, G Reaven, and J Olefsky. "Postprandial plasma-glucose and insulin responses to different complex carbohydrates," *Diabetes* 26 (1977): 1178–1183.

Credit, Larry P, OMD, Sharon G. Hartunian, LICSW, and Margaret J. Nowak, CMT. *Your Guide to Complementary Medicine.* Garden City Park, NY: Avery Publishing Group, 1998.

Cunningham-Rundles, S, ed. *Nutrient Modulation of the Immune Response.* New York, NY: Marcel Deckker, 1993.

Dagnelie, PC. "Some algae are potentially adequate sources of vitamin B_{12}," *Journal of Nutrition* 127(2) (1997): 379.

D'Amico G, et al. "Effect of vegetarian soy diet on hyperlipidemia in nephrotic syndrome," *Lancet* 339 (1992): 1131–1134.

Daniel, R. "Research on diets and cancer strong enough to prompt action," *Nursing Times* 90(3) (1994): 23.

Darnton, J. "Britain Admits Link of 'Mad-Cow' Disease to Humans," *New York Times,* March 21, 1996.

Dawson-Hughes, B, et al. "Rates of bone loss in postmenopausal women randomly assigned to one of two dosages of vitamin D," *American Journal of Clinical Nutrition* 61(5) (1995): 1140–1145.

Debry, G. "Diet peculiarities. Vegetarianism, veganism, crudivorism, macrobiotism," *Rev Prat* 41(11) (1991): 967–972.

DelToma, E, et al. "Soluble and insoluble dietary fibre in diabetic diets," *European Journal of Clinical Nutrition* 42 (1988): 313–319.

Denver, MB. "Maximum milk output defended growth hormone a hot issue," *Denver Post* (Dec 20, 1994): A–1.

Diamond, W John, MD, W Lee Cowden, MD, with Burton Goldberg. *An Alternative Medicine Guide to Cancer.* Tiburon, CA: Future Medicine Publishing, Inc., 1997.

"Dietary status of Seventh Day Adventist vegetarian and non-vegetarian elderly women," *Journal of the American Medical Association* 89 (1989): 1763–1769.

Doll, R, and R Peto. *The Causes of Cancer.* New York, NY: Oxford University Press, 1981.

Dong, A, and SC Scott. "Serum vitamin B_{12} and blood cell values in vegetarians," *Annals of Nutrition and Metabolism* 26(4) (1982): 209–216.

Donovan, UM, and RS Givson. "Dietary intakes of adolescent females consuming vegetarian, semi-vegetarian, and omnivorous diets," *Journal of Adolescent Health* 18(4) (1996): 292–300.

Donovan, UM, and RS Givson. "Iron and zinc status of young women aged 14 to 19 years consuming vegetarian and omnivorous diets," *Journal of the American College of Nutrition* 14(5) (1995): 463–472.

Drajcovicove-Kudlackove, M, et al. "Biochemial and hematologic indicators in the blood of young vegetarians," *Bratisl Lek Listy* 94(12) (1993): 621–625.

Durning, AT, and HB Brough. *Taking stock: animal farming and the environment.* Washington, DC: Worldwatch Institute, 1991: Worldwatch Paper 103.

Duyff, Roberta L. *The American Dietetic Association's Complete Food and Nutrition Guide.* Minneapolis, MN: Chronimed Publishing, 1998.

Draper, A, et al. "The energy and nutrient intakes of different types of vegetarians: a case for supplements?", *British Journal of Nutrition* 69(1) (1993): 3–19.

Dwyer, JT. "Health aspects of vegetarian diets," *American Journal of Clinical Nutrition* 48(suppl 3) (1988): 12–38.

Dwyer, JT. "Nutritional consequences of vegetarianism," *Annual Review of Nutrition* 11 (1991): 61–91.

Easterling, TR, and TJ Benedetti. "Preeclampsia: A hyperdynamic disease model," *American Journal of Obstetrics & Gynecology* 160 (1989): 1447–1453.

Eisenstein, Phyllis, and Samuel M Scheiner, PhD. *Overcoming the Pain of Inflammatory Arthritis: The Pain-Free Promise of Pantothenic Acid.* Garden City Park, NY: Avery Publishing Group, 1997.

Eisinger, M, et al. "Nutrient intake of endurance runners with ovo-lactovegetarian diet and regular western diet," *Zeitschrift fur Ernahrungswessenschaft* 33(3) (1994): 217–229.

Ellis, FR. "The nutritional status of vegans and vegetarians," *Symposium Proceedings* 26 (1969): 205–211.

Ellis, FR, S Holesh, and JW Ellis. "Incidence of osteoporosis in vegetarians and omnivores," *American Journal of Clinical Nutrition* 25 (1972): 555–558.

Ellis, FR, and VM Montegriffo. "Veganism, clinical findings and investigations," *American Journal of Clinical Nutrition* 23(30) (1970): 249–255.

Environmental Protection Agency. *EPA Workgroup Report,* 1994, cited in Jim Mason's "Fowling the Waters," *E Magazine* (Sept/Oct 1995): 33.

Epstein, SS. "The chemical jungle: Today's beef industry," *International Journal of Health Services* 20(2) (1990): 277–280.

Etherton, K, et al. "The effect of diet on plasma lipids, lipoproteins, and coronary heart disease," *Journal of the American Dietetic Association* 88 (1988): 1373–1400.

Evans, WJ, and D Cyr-Campbell. "Nutrition, exercise, and healthy aging," *Journal of the American Dietetic Association* 97(6) (1997): 632–638.

Expert Panel on Detection, Evaluation, and Treatment of High Blood Cholesterol in Adults. "Summary of the Second Report of the Nation Cholesterol Education Program (NCEP) Expert Panel, National Cholesterol Education Program on Detection, Evaluation, and Treatment of High Blood Cholesterol In Adults (Adult Treatment Panel II)," *Journal of the American Medical Association* 269(23) (1993): 3015–3023.

Falak, Frank, MD, PhD. "Why?", www.mojones.com/mother_jones/MJ94/castleman.html, (1998).

Finley, DA, et al. "Food choices of vegetarians and nonvegetarians during pregnancy and lactation," *Journal of the American Dietetic Association* 85(6) (1985): 678–685.

Finn, SC. "Women in the new world order: Where old values command new respect," *Journal of the American Dietetic Association* 97(5) (1997): 475–480.

Fisher, H, and E Boe. *The Rutger's Guide to Lowering Your Cholesterol.* New Brunswick, NJ: Rutgers University Press, 1985.

Fisher, M, et al. "The effect of vegetarian diet on plasma lipid and platelet levels," *Archives of Internal Medicine* 146(6) (1986): 193–197.

Fonnebo, V. "Mortality in Norwegian Seventh Day Adventist 1962–1986," *Journal of Clinical Epidemiology* 45(2) (1992): 157–167.

Fonnebo, V. "The Tromso Heart Study: Diet, religion, and risk factor for coronary heart disease," *American Journal of Clinical Nutrition* 48 (1988): 826–829.

Fotsis, T, et al. "Genistein, a dietary-derived inhibitor of in vitro angiogenesis," *Proceedings of the National Academy of Sciences of the United States of America* 90(7) (1993): 2690–2694.

Fraser, GE. "Determinants of ischemic heart disease in Seventh-Day Adventists: a review," *American Journal of Clinical Nutrition* 48 (1988): 833–836.

Fraser, GE. "Diet and coronary heart disease: beyond dietary fats and low-density lipoprotein cholesterol," *American Journal of Clinical Nutrition* 59(suppl) (1994): 1122–1123s.

Fraser, GE, et al. "A possible protective effect of nut consumption on risk of coronary heart disease," *Archives of Internal Medicine* 152 (1992): 1416–1424.

Fraser, GE, WL Beeson, and RL Phillips. "Diet and lung cancer in California Seventh Day Adventists," *American Journal of Epidemiology* 133(7) (1991): 683–693.

Fraser, GE, KD Lindsted, and WL Beeson. "Effect of risk factor values on lifetime risk of and age at first coronary event: The Adventist Health Study," *American Journal of Epidemiology* 142(7) (1995): 746–758.

Freeland-Graves, JH. "Mineral adequacy of vegetarian diets," *American Journal of Clinical Nutrition* 48(suppl 3) (1988): 859–862.

Freeland-Graves, JH, PW Bodzy, and ML Ebangit. "Zinc and copper content of foods used in vegetarian diets," *Journal of the American Dietetic Association* 77(6) (1980): 648–654.

Freeland-Graves, JH, PW Bodzy, and MA Epright. "Zinc status of vegetarians," *Journal of the American Dietetic Association* 77(6) (1980): 648–654.

Frentzel-Beyme R, and Claude J Chang. "Vegetarian diets and colon cancer: the German experience," *American Journal of Clinical Nutrition* 59(suppl 5) (1994): 1143s–1152s.

Frentzel-Beyme R, Claude J Chang, and G Eilber. "Mortality among German vegetarians: First results after five years of follow-up," *Nutrition and Cancer* 11(2) (1988): 117–126.

Fries, GF, and GS Marrow. "Excretion of polybrominated biphenyls into the milk of cows," *Journal of Dairy Science* 58(6) (1975): 947–951.

Gallenberg, LA, and MJ Vodicnik. "Transfer of persistent chemicals in milk," *Drug Metabolism Reviews* 21(2) (1989): 277–317.

Garritson, BK, et al. "The effect of diet changes on the immune system of breast cancer patients," *Cancer Researcher Weekly* (Nov 22, 1993): 18.

Gastelu, Daniel, and Fred Hatfield, PhD. *Dynamic Nutrition for Maximum Performance: A Complete Nutritional Guide for Peak Sports Performance.* Garden City Park, NY: Avery Publishing Group, 1997.

Geil, PB. "The 1994 Nutrition Recommendations for Diabetes: Is Fiber a Factor?", *Soy Connection* 3(2) (1995): 2.

Ghosh, J, and S Das. "Evaluation of vitamin A and C status in normal and malignant conditions and their possible role in cancer prevention," *Japanese Journal of Cancer Research* 76 (1985): 1174–1178.

Giacoia, GP, C Catz, and SJ Yaffe. "Environmental hazards in milk and infant nutrition," *Clinical Obstetrics & Gynecology* 26(2) (1983): 458–466.

Giehl, Dudley. "Vegetarianism, a way of life," from *Encyclopedia Americana* (vol 27). New York, NY: Harper and Row, 1979.

Giem, P, WL Beeson, and GE Fraser. "The incidence of dementia and intake of animal products: preliminary findings from the Adventist Health Study," *Neuroepidemiology* 12(1) (1993): 28–36.

Giovannucci, E, et al. "Relation of diet to the risk of colorectal adenoma in men," *Journal of the National Cancer Institute* 84(1992): 91–98.

Glore, SR, et al. "Soluable fiber and serum lipids: a literature review," *Journal of the American Dietetic Association* 94 (1994): 425–436.

Golbitz, P. "Traditional soyfoods: processing and products," *Journal of Nutrition* 125(suppl 3) (1995): 570s–572s.

Goldberg, MJ, JW Smith, and RL Nichols. "Comparison of the fecal microflora of Seventh-Day Adventists with individuals consuming a general diet. Implications concerning colonic carcinoma," *Annals of Surgery* 186(1) (1977): 97–100.

Goldfarb, S. "The role of diet in the pathogenesis and therapy of nephrolithiesis," *Endocrinology and Metabolism Clinics of North America* 19(4) (Dec, 1990): 805–820.

Gorbach, SL. "Estrogens, breast cancer, and intestinal flora," *Reviews of Infectious Diseases* 6(suppl 1) (1984): S85–90.

Gordan, Dennis. "Eating Green," *Diabetes Forecast* (Mar, 1995): 36–42, 81–84.

Graf, E, and JW Eaton. "Antioxidant functions of phytic acid," *Free Radical Biology and Medicine* 8(1) (1990): 61–69.

Graham, SM, OM Arvela, and GA Wise. "Long-term neurologic consequences of nutritional vitamin B_{12} deficiency in infants," *Journal of Pediatrics* 121 (1992): 710–714.

Gretz, N, E Melsinger, and M Strauch. "Influence of diet and underlying renal disease on the rate of progression of chronic renal failure," *Infusionstherapie und Klinische Ernahrung* 12(suppl 5) (1987): 21–25.

Griffith, HW. *Vitamins, Herbs, Minerals & Supplements.* Tucson, AZ: Fisher Books, 1988.

Grundy, SM, and GL Vega. "Two different views of the relationship of hyperglyceridemia to coronary heart disease," *Archives of Internal Medicine* 152 (1992): 2834.

"Guest Editorial: A new nutritional approach in cancer therapy in light of mechanistic understanding of cancer causation and development," *Journal of the American College of Nutrition* 12(3) (1993): 205–208.

Gursche, Siegfried, MH. *Encyclopedia of National Healing.* Zoltan Rona, med. ed. Blaine, WA: National Life Publishing, Inc., 1997.

Gussow, JD. "Ecology and vegetarian considerations: does environmental responsibility demand the elimination of livestock?", *American Journal of Clinical Nutrition* 59 (suppl) (1994): 1110s–1116s.

Gwinn, R, et al. *The Encyclopaedia Brittanica* (vol 12). Chicago, IL: 1989.

Haddad, EH. "Development of a vegetarian food guide," *American Journal of Clinical Nutrition* 59(suppl) (1994): 1248s–1254s.

Hager, Dr., and Linda Hager. *Stress and the Woman's Body.* Fleming H. Revell, Co., 1998.

Handler, S. "Dietary fiber: Can it prevent certain colonic diseases?", *Postgraduate Medicine* 73(2) (1983): 301–307.

Hankin, JH, and V Rawlings. "Diet and breast cancer: A Review," *American Journal of Clinical Nutrition* 31: 2005–2016.

Hasley, William, ed., et al. *Colliers Encyclopedia* (vol 23). New York, NY: Macmillan, 1974.

Hausman, Patricia. *Right Dose: How to Take Vitamins and Minerals Safely.* New York, NY: Ballantine Books, 1989.

Havala, S, and J Dwyer. "Position of the American Dietetic Association: Vegetarian Diets," *Journal of the American Dietetic Association* 88(3) (1988): 352–355.

Havala S, and J Dwyer. "Position of the American Dietetic Association: Vegetarian Diets," *Journal of the American Dietetic Association* 93(11) (1993): 1317–1319.

Heaney, RP. "Calcium supplements: practical considerations," *Osteoporosis International* 1 (1991): 65–71.

Heaney, RP, and RR Recker. "Effects of nitrogen, phosphorus, and caffeine on calcium balance in women," *Journal of Laboratory and Clinical Medicine* 92 (1982): 741–743.

Heber, David, MD, PhD. *The Resolution Diet.* Garden City Park, NY: Avery Publishing Group, 1999.

Hegarty, PVJ. "Nutrition and health factors in meat consumption," *Journal of Animal Science* 48(2) (1979): 408–413.

Hegsted, M, et al. "Urinary calcium and calcium balance in young men as affected by level of protein and phosphorus intake," *Journal of Nutrition* 111 (1981): 553–562.

Helman, AD, and I Darnton-Hill. "Vitamin and iron status in new vegetarians," *American Journal of Clinical Nutrition* 45(4) (1987): 785–789.

Herbert, V. "Staging vitamin B_{12} (cobalamin) status in vegetarians," *American Journal of Clinical Nutrition* 59(suppl 5) (1994): 1213s–1222s.

Herbert, V. "Vitamin B_{12}: plant sources, requirements, and assay," *American Journal of Clinical Nutrition* 48(suppl 3) (1988): 852–858.

Hill, P, et al. "Environmental factors and breast and prostatic cancer," *Cancer Research* 41(9, pt 2) (1981): 3817–3818.

Hill, P, et al. "Peptide and steroid hormones in subjects at different risk for diet-related diseases," *American Journal of Clinical Nutrition* 48(suppl 3) (1988): 782–786.

Hill, PB, and EL Wynder. "Effect of a vegetarian diet and dexamethasone on plasma prolactin, testosterone and dehydroepiandrosterone in men and women," *Cancer Letters* 7(5) (1979): 273–282.

Hirayma, T. "Mortality in Japanese with lifestyles similar to Seventh Day Adventists: Strategy for risk reduction by lifestyle modification," *National Cancer Institute Monographs* 69 (1985): 143–153.

Hoffman, Goetz L, and BK Pedersen. "Exercise and the immune system: a model of the stress response?", *Immunology Today* 15(8) (1994): 382–387.

Holl, MG, and LH Allen. "Comparative effects of meals high in protein, sucrose, or starch on human mineral metabolism and insulin secretion," *American Journal of Clinical Nutrition* 48(5) (1988): 1219–1225.

Hostmark, AT, et al. "Reduced plasma fibrinogen, serum, peroxides, lipids, and apolipoproteins after a 3-week vegetarian diet," *Plant Foods for Human Nutrition* 43(1) (1993): 55–61.

Howie, BJ, and TD Shultz. "Dietary and hormonal interrelationships among vegetarian Seventh Day Adventist and nonvegetarian men," *American Journal of Clinical Nutrition* 42(1) (1985): 127–134.

Huang, CT, GS Gopalakrishna, and BL Nichols. "Fiber, intestinal sterols, and colon cancer," *American Journal of Clinical Nutrition* 31(3) (1978): 515–526.

Hughes, H, and TAB Sanders. "Riboflavin levels in the diet and breast milk of vegans and omnivores," *Proceedings of the Nutrition Society* 38(2) (1979): 95A.

Hunt, IF, et al. "Bone mineral content in post-menopausal women: Comparison of omnivores and vegetarians," *American Journal of Clinical Nutrition* 50 (1989): 517–523.

Hunt, IF, NJ Murphy, and C Henderson. "Food and nutrient intake of Seventh Day Adventist women," *American Journal of Clinical Nutrition* 48(3) (1988): 850–851.

Groff, James, Sareen Gropper, and Sara Hunt. *Advanced Nutrition and Human Metabolism.* Belmont, CA: West/Wadsworth, 1995.

Hunter, DJ, et al. "A prospective study on the intake of vitamins C, E, and A and the risk of breast cancer," *New England Journal of Medicine* 329 (1993): 234–240.

Hunter, JE. "Omega-3 Fatty acids from vegetable oils," *American Journal of Clinical Nutrition* 51(5) (1990): 809–814.

Hutchinson, Karen Anne, MD, and Judith Sachs. *What Every Woman Needs to Know About Estrogen: National and Traditional Therapies for a Longer, Healthier Life.* New York, NY: Plume, 1997.

Immermman. "Vitamin B_{12} status on a vegetarian diet," *World Review of Nutrition and Dietetics* 37 (1981): 38–54.

Indiana Soybean Board. *US 1998 Soyfoods Directory.* Lebanon, IN: Indiana Soybean Board, 1998.

Inglis, Les. *Diet for a Gentle World: Eating With Conscience.* Garden City Park, NY: Avery Publishing Group, 1993.

Ingram, DM. "Trends in diet and breast cancer mortality in England and Wales," *Nutrition & Cancer* 3(2) (1981): 75–80.

Ito, H, et al. "Evaluation of diet of calcium stone patients" (in Japanese), *Hinyokiki Kiyo-Acta Urologica Japnica* 38(1, abstract) (1992): 9–14.

Jacobs, C, and JT Dwyer. "Vegetarian children: appropriate and inappropriate diets," *American Journal of Clinical Nutrition* 48 (1988): 811–818.

Jacobs, L. *Waste of the West: Public Lands Ranching.* Tucson, AZ: Lynn Jacobs, 1991.

Jacobson, MF, LY Lefferts, and AW Garland. *Safe Food: Eating Wisely in a Risky World.* Living Planet Press, 1991.

Janelle, KC, and SI Barr. "Nutrient intakes and eating behaviour scores of vegetarian and non-vegetarian women," *Journal of the American Dietetic Association* 95 (1995): 180–186, 189.

Jansson, B. "Geographic cancer risk and intracellular potassium and sodium ratios," *Cancer Detection and Prevention* 9(304) (1986): 171–194.

Jenkins, DJA, et al. "Glycemic index of foods: A physiological basis for carbohydrate exchange," *American Journal of Clinical Nutrition* 34 (1981): 362–366.

Jensen, Dr. Bernard, and Mark Anderson. *Empty Harvest: Understanding the Link Between Our Food, Our Immunity, & Our Planet.* Garden City Park, NY: Avery Publishing Group, 1990.

Jibani, MM, et al. "Predominantly vegetarian diet in patients with incipient and early clinical diabetic nephropathy: effects on albumin excretion rate and nutritional status," *Diabetes Medicine* 8(10) (1991): 949–953.

Johnsen, JB, and V Fonnebo. "Vitamin B_{12} deficiency in strict vegetarian diet. Why do some people choose such a diet, and what will they do in the case of vitamin B_{12} deficiency?", *Tidsskrify for den Norske Laegeforening* 111(1) (1991): 62–64.

Johnsen, JM, and PM Walker. "Zinc and iron utilization in young women consuming a beef-based diet," *Journal of the American Dietetic Association* 92(12) (1992): 1474–1478.

Johnson, ES, et al. "Occurrence of cancer in women in the meat industry," *British Journal of Industrial Medicine* 43(9) (1986): 597–604.

Johnson, NE, EN Alcantra, and H Linkswiler. "Effect of level of protein intake on urinary and fecal calcium retention of young males," *Journal of Nutrition* 100 (1970): 1425–1430.

Johnston, PK, E Haddad, and J Sabvate. "The vegetarian adolescent," in MP Nussbaum and JT Dwyer's (ed.) *Adolescent medicine: state of the art reviews.* Philadelphia, PA: Hanley & Belfus, no 3, 1992: 417–437.

Journal of the American Dietetic Association 97(11) (1997): 1317–1321.

Kaneda, N, C Nagata, M Kabuto, et al. "Fat and fiber intakes in relation to serum estrogen concentration in pre-menopausal Japanese women," *Nutrition and Cancer* 27 (1997): 279–283.

Kaplan, NM. "Dietary aspects of the treatment of hypertension," *Annual Review of Public Health* 7 (1986): 503–519.

Karisson, J, et al. "Predictors and effects of long-term dieting on mental well-being and weight loss in obese women," *Appetite* 23(1) (1994): 15–26.

Katan, MB, and RP Mensink. "Isomeric Fatty Acids and Serum Lipoproteins," *Nutrition Reviews* 50(4) (1992): 46–48.

Kay, K. "Polybrominated biphenyls (PBB) environmental contamination in Michigan, 1973–1976," *Environmental Research* 13(1) (1977): 74–93.

Key, TJ, et al. "Dietary habits and mortality in 11,000 vegetarians and health conscious people: results of a 17-year follow-up," *British Medical Journal* 313(7060) (1996): 775–779.

Khansari, DN, AJ Murgo, and RE Faith. "Effects of stress on the immune system," *Immunology Today* 11(5) (1990): 170–175.

King, JC, T Stein, and M Doyle. "Effect of vegetarianism on the zinc status of pregnant women," *American Journal of Clinical Nutrition* 34 (1981): 1049–1055.

Kinsella, JE. "Reply to O Odeleye and R Watson," *American Journal of Clinical Nutrition* 53 (1991): 178.

Kjeldsen-Kragh, J, et al. "Controlled trial of fasting and one year vegetarian diet in rheumatoid arthritis," *Lancet* 338(8772) (1991): 899–902.

Kjeldsen-Kragh, J, et al. "Vegetarian diet for patients with rheumatoid arthritis: can the clinical effects be explained by the psychological characteristics of the patients?", *British Journal of Rheumatology* 33(6) (1994): 569–575.

Kjeldsen-Kragh, J, et al. "Vegetarian diet for patients with rheumatoid arthritis status: two years after introduction of the diet," *Clinical Rheumatology* 13(3) (1994): 475–482.

Klockenbrink, M. "The New Range War Has the Desert as Foe," *New York Times,* August 20, 1991: C4.

Knutsen, SF, et al. "Lifestyle and the use of health services," *American Journal of Clinical Nutrition* 59(suppl) (1994): 1171s–1175s.

Korpela, JT, H Adlercreutz, and MJ Turunen. "Fecal free and conjugated bile acids and neutral sterols in vegetarians, omnivores, and patients with colorectal cancer," *Scandinavian Journal of Gastroenterology* 23(3) (1988): 277–283.

Krajcovicova-Kudlackova, M, et al. "Lipid and pro-oxidative and antioxidative parameters in the blood of vegetarians," *Bratisl Lek Listy* 95(8) (1994): 344–348.

Krajcovicova-Kudlackova, M, et al. "Lipid parameters in blood of vegetarians," *Cor Vasa* 35(6) (1993): 224–229.

Krajcovicova-Kudlackova, M, et al. "Selected parameters of lipid metabolism in young vegetarians," *Annals of Nutrition Metabolism* 38(6) (1994): 331–335.

Kramer, LB, et al. "Mineral and trace element content of vegetarian diets," *Journal of the American College of Nutrition* 3(1) (1984): 3–11.

Krauss, RM, et al. "Dietary Guidelines for Healthy American Adults," *Circulation* 94 (1996): 1795–1800.

Kris-Etherton, PM, et al. "The effect of diet on plasma lipids, lipoproteins, and coronary heart disease," *Journal of the American Dietetic Association* 88(11) (1988): 1373–1400.

Kris-Etherton, PM, and SS Jonnalagadola. "The role of soybean oil in diets that reduce cardiovascular disease risk," *Soy Connection* 4(2) (1996): 1.

Kritchevsky, D, SA Tepper, and G Goodman. "Diet, nutrition intake, and metabolism in populations at high and low risk for colon cancer. Relationship of diet to serum lipids," *American Journal of Clinical Nutrition* 40 (suppl 4) (1984): 921–929.

Krizmaric, J. "Here's Who We Are," *Vegetarian Times* (Oct, 1992): 72.

Kuhne, T, R Bubl, and R Baumgartner. "Maternal vegan diet causing a serious infantile neurological disorder due to vitamin B_{12} deficiency," *European Journal of Pediatrics* 150(3) (1991): 205–208.

Kulkarni, K. "Soy: The Perfect Protein," *Diabetes Self-Management* (Sept/Oct, 1996): 32–36.

Kumpusalo, E, et al. "Multivitamin supplementation of adult omnivores and lacto-vegetarians: circulation levels of vitamin A, D, and E, lipids, apolipoproteins and selenium," *International Journal for Vitamin and Nutrition Research* 60(1) (1990): 58–66.

Kunkel, ME, and RE Beauchene. "Protein intake and urinary excretion of protein-derived metabolites in aging female vegetarians and nonvegetarians," *Journal of the American College of Nutrition* 10(4) (1991): 308–314.

Kurup, PA, et al. "Diet, nutrition intake and metabolism in populations at high and low risk for colon cancer: composition, intake, and excretion of fiber constituents," *American Journal of Clinical Nutrition* 40(suppl 4) (1984): 942–946.

Kushi, LH, EB Lenart, and WC Willett. "Health implications of Mediterranean diets in light of contemporary knowledge: Meat, wine, fats, oils," *American Journal of Clinical Nutrition* 61(suppl) (1995): 1416s–1427s.

Lafferty, MB, and S Powers. "Dioxin: How Much Is Out There?", *Columbus Dispatch* (1994): 5f.

Lappé, Frances Moore. *Diet for a Small Planet.* New York, NY: Ballantine Books, Inc., 1971.

Lappé, Frances Moore. *Diet for a Small Planet.* New York, NY: Ballantine Books, Inc., 1982.

Lark, Susan M, MD. *Menstrual Cramps: A Self-Help Program.* Los Altos, CA: Westchester Publishing Company, 1993.

Lark, Susan M, MD. *The Estrogen Decision: A Self-Help Book.* Berkeley, CA: Celestial Arts, 1996.

LaVecchia, C, et al. "A case-control study of diet and gastric cancer in Northern Italy," *International Journal of Cancer* 40 (1987): 484–489.

Lee, G. "EPA study links dioxin to cancer: report stops short of calling chemical a known carcinogen," *Washington Post,* September 12, 1994: a1.

Levin, N, J Rattan, and T Gilat. "Energy intake and body weight in ovo-lactovegetarians," *Journal of Clinical Gastroenterology* 8(4) (1986): 451–453.

Levenstein, Mary Kerney. *Everyday Cancer Risks and How to Avoid Them.* Garden City Park, NY: Avery Publishing Group, 1992.

Lewis, S. "An opinion on the global impact of meat consumption," *American Journal of Clinical Nutrition* 59(suppl) (1994): 1099s–1102s.

Lieberman, Shari, PhD, and Nancy Bruning. *The Real Vitamin and Mineral Book: Using Supplements for Optimum Health* (2nd ed). Garden City Park, NY: Avery Publishing Group, 1997.

Lighttowler, HJ, GJ Davies, and MD Trevan. "Iodine in the diet: perspectives for vegans," *Journal of the Royal Society of Health* 116(1) (1996): 14–20.

Lindalh, O, et al. "A vegan regimen with reduced medication in the treatment of hypertension," *British Journal of Nutrition* 52(1) (1984): 11–20.

Ling, WH, and O Hanninen. "Shifting from a conventional diet to an uncooked vegan diet reversibly alters fecal hydrolytic activities in humans," *Journal of Nutrition* 122(4) (1992): 924–930.

Lipkin, M, et al. "Seventh Day Adventist vegetarians have a quiescent proliferative activity in colonic mucosa," *Cancer Letters* 26(2) (1985): 139–144.

"Livingston-Wheeler Therapy," *A Cancer Journal for Clinicians* 40(2) (1990): 103–108.

Lloyd, T, et al. "Urinary hormonal concentrations and spinal bone densities of premenopausal vegetarian and nonvegetarian women," *American Journal of Clinical Nutrition* 50 (1989): 517–523.

Lowik, MR, et al. "Effect of dietary fiber on the vitamin B_6 status among vegetarian and nonvegetarian elderly (Dutch Nutrition Surveillance System)," *Journal of the American College of Nutrition* 9(3) (1990): 241–249.

Lowik, MR, et al. "Long-term effects of vegetarian diet on the nutritional status of elderly people (Dutch Nutrition Surveillance System)," *Journal of the American College of Nutrition* 9(6) (1990): 600–609.

Mackinnon, LT. "Current challenges and future expectations in exercise immunology: back to the future," *Medicine & Science in Sports & Exercise* 26(2) (1994): 191–194.

Mandel, CH, et al. "Dietary intake and plasma concentrations of vitamin E, vitamin C, and beta carotene in patients with coronary artery diseases," *Journal of the American Dietetic Association* 97(6) (1997): 655–657.

Malter, M, G Schriever, and U Eilber. "Natural killer cells, vitamins, and other blood components of vegetarian and omnivorous man," *Nutrition Cancer* 12(3) (1989): 271–278.

Marangella, M, et al. "Effect of animal and vegetable protein intake on oxalate excretion in idopathic calcium stone disease," *British Journal of Urology* 63(4) (1989): 348–351.

Marcus, MB. "Turkey à la microbes?", *U.S. News and World Report* 123(20) (1997): 79.

Margetts, BM, et al. "Vegetarian diet in mild hypertension: A randomized controlled trial," *British Medical Journal of Clinical Research and Education* 293(6560) (1986): 1468–1471.

Margetts, BM, et al. "Vegetarian diet in mild hypertension: Effects of fat and fiber," *American Journal of Clinical Nutrition* 48 (suppl 3) (1988): 801–805.

Marino, DD, and JC King. "Nutritional concerns during adolescence," *Pediatric Clinics of North America* 27(1) (1980): 125–139.

March, AG, et al. "Coritcal bone density of adult lacto-ovovegetarian and omnivorous women," *Journal of the American Dietetic Association* 80(6) (1980): 148–155.

Marsh, AG, et al. "Vegetarian lifestyle and bone mineral density," *American Journal of Clinical Nutrition* 48 (1988): 837–841.

Martinez, L. *The Complete Juicer.* Philadelphia, PA: Running Press, 1992.

Maruchi, N, et al. "Relation of food consumption to cancer mortality in Japan with special reference to international figures," *Gann* 68(1) (1977): 1–13.

Masarci, JR, et al. "Vegetarian diets, lipids and cardiovascular risk," *Australia and New Zealand Journal of Medicine* 14(4) (1984): 400–404.

Mason, J. "Fowling the Waters," *E Magazine* (Sept/Oct, 1995): 33.

Mason, J, and P Singer. *Animal Factories.* New York: Harmony Books, 1990.

Massey, LK, and SJ Whiting. "Dietary salt, urinary calcium, and bone loss," *Journal of Bone Mineral Research* 11 (1996): 731–736.

Mather, A. "Elvira's Halloween Hints," *Vegetarian Times* 230 (1996): 136.

Mazess, RB, and W Mather. "Bone mineral content of North Alaskan Eskimos," *American Journal of Clinical Nutrition* 27 (1974): 916–925.

McDougall, J, et al. "Rapid reduction of serum cholesterol and blood pressure by a twelve-day, very low fat, strictly vegetarian diet," *Journal of the American College of Nutrition* 14(5) (1995): 491–496.

McGinn, KA, and PJ Haylock. *Women's Cancers: How to Prevent Them, How to Treat Them, How to Beat Them.* Alameda, CA: Hunter House, Inc., 1998.

McKeigue, PM, et al. "Diet and fecal steroid profile in a South Asian population with a low colon-cancer rate," *American Journal of Clinical Nutrition* 50(1) (1989): 151–154.

McNeill, DA, PS Ali, and YS Song. "Mineral analyses of vegetarian, health and conventional foods: magnesium, zinc, copper, and manganese content," *Journal of the American Dietetic Association* 85 (1985): 569–573.

Medkova, IL, et al. "Balanced vegetarian diet in combined rehabilitation of patients suffering from ischemic heart diseases," *Klinicheskaia Meditsina* 75(1) (1997): 28–31.

Medkova, IL, et al. "Feasibility of correcting lipid metabolism in patients with cardiovascular diseases using a balanced vegetarian diet," *Voprosy Pitannia* 2 (1996): 29–32.

Melby, CL, DG Goldflied, and ML Toohey. "Blood pressure differences in older black and white long-term vegetarians and nonvegetarians," *Journal of the American College of Nutrition* 12(3) (1993): 262–269.

Melby, CL, ML Toohey, and J Cebrick. "Blood pressure and blood lipids among vegetarian, semivegetarian, and nonvegetarian African Americans," *American Journal of Clinical Nutrition* 59(1) (1994): 103–109.

Melchert, HU, et al. "Fatty acid patterns in triglycerides, diglycerides, free fatty acids, cholesteryl esters and phosphatidylcholine in serum from vegetarians and non-vegetarians," *Atherosclerosis* 65 (1–2) (1987): 159–166.

Menger, RG, et al. "Dietary assessment of older Iowa women with a food frequency questionnaire: nutrient intake, reproductibility, and comparison with 24-hour dietary recall interviews," *American Journal of Epidemiology* 136(1992): 192–200.

Messena, M, JW Erdman Jr, eds. "First international symposium on the role of soy in preventing and treating chronic disease," *Journal of Nutrition* 125(suppl) (1995): 567s–808s.

Messina, MJ. "Diet, soy and heart disease prevention," *Soy Connection* 3(3) (1995): 1.

Messina, MJ. "Osteoporosis—not just a deficiency disease," *Soy Connection* 2(2) (1997): 1, 2.

Messina, MJ. "Thoughts on dietary fat—requirements and optimal amounts," *Soy Connection* 4(2) (1996): 1.

Messina, MJ. "A viable alternative to drug approach," *Soy Connection* 4(1) (1996): 2.

Messina, MJ, AG Patterson, and CB Bearden. "Researchers from around the world present on wide range of chronic diseases," *Soy Connection* 5(1) (1997): 1–4.

Metz, JA, JJ Anderson, and PN Gallagher Jr. "Intakes of calcium, phosphorus, and protein, and physical-activity level are related to radial bone mass in young adult women," *American Journal of Clinical Nutrition* 58(4) (1993): 537–542.

Meydani, SN, et al. "Vitamin E supplementation and in vivo immune response in healthy elderly subjects," *Journal of the American Medical Association* 277 (1997): 1380–1386.

Mills, KD, et al. "Bladder cancer in a low risk population: Results from the Adventist Health Study," *American Journal of Epidemiology* 133(3) (1991): 230–239.

Mills, KD, et al. "Cancer incidence among California Seventh Day Adventists 1976–1982," *American Journal of Clinical Nutrition* 59(suppl) (1994): 1136s–1142s.

Mills, KD, et al. "Dietary habits and breast cancer incidence among Seventh Day Adventists," *Cancer* 64(3) (1989): 582–590.

Mirkin, G. "Walnuts and serum lipids," *New England Journal of Medicine* 329(5) (1993): 358.

Miruish, SS. "Effects of vitamins C and E on N-nitroso compound formation, carcinogenesis, and cancer," *Cancer* 158L (1986): 1842–1850.

Morgan, SA, K O'Dea, and AJ Sinclair. "A low-fat diet supplemented with monounsaturated fat results in less HDL-D lowering than a very low fat diet," *Journal of the American Dietetic Association* 97(2) (1997): 151–156.

Must, A, et al. "Long-term morbidity and mortality of overweight adolescents: a follow-up of the Harvard Growth Study of 1922 to 1935," *New England Journal of Medicine* 327 (1992): 1350–1356.

Mutch, PB. "Food guides for the vegetarian," *American Journal of Clinical Nutrition* 48 (1988): 913–919.

Myers, N. *The Primary Source: Tropical Forests and Our Future* (1992) in L Brown et al's *Vital Signs 1994*, Washington DC: Worldwatch Institute, 1994: 32.

Nair, P, et al. "Diet, nutrition intake, and metabolism in populations at high and low risk of colon cancer. Metabolism of neutral sterols," *American Journal of Clinical Nutrition* 40 (suppl 4) (1984): 931–936.

Nair, P, and JF Mayberry. "Vegetarianism, dietary fiber and gastro-intestinal diseases," *Digestive Diseases* 12(3) (1994): 177–185.

Naissmith, BJ, SK Rana, and PW Emery. "Metabolism of taurine during reproduction in women," *Human Nutrition: Clinical Nutrition* 40c (1986): 37–45.

National Dairy Council. "Dietary Reference Intakes: Calcium and related nutrients," *Dairy Council Digest* 68(6) (1997): 31–36.

National Health and Medical Research Council. *Report of the Working Party on Sodium in the Australian Diet.* Canberra, Australia: Australian Government Publishing Service, 1984.

National Institutes of Health. *Understanding Adult Obesity.* Bethesda, MD: National Institutes of Health.

National Research Council. *Diet and Health: Implications for Reducing Chronic Diseases Risk.* Washington, DC: National Academy Press, 1989.

National Research Council. *Recommended Dietary Allowances* (10th ed). Washington, DC: National Academy Press, 1989.

Nations, JD, and DI Komer. "Rainforests and the hamburger society," *Environment* 25 (1983): 12–20.

Natural Resources Defense Council and International Alliance for Sustainable Agriculture. *Hog Wash: Factory Farm Giveaways in Clean Water Act Proposals.* New York, NY: Natural Resources Defense Council and International Alliance for Sustainable Agriculture: July, 1995.

Nelson, M, F Bakaliou, and A Trivedi. "Iron-deficiency anaemia and physical performance in adolescent girls from different ethnic backgrounds," *British Journal of Nutrition* 72(3) (1994): 427–433.

New England Journal of Medicine 323 (1990): 439.

Newcomer, AD. "Lactase deficiency," *Contemporary Nutrition* 4 (1979): 1–2.

Nieman, DC, et al. "Dietary status of Seventh Day-Adventist vegetarian and non-vegetarian elderly women," *Journal of the American Dietetic Association* 89(12) (1989): 1763–1769.

Nieman, DC, et al. "Hematological, anthropometric, and metabolic comparisons between vegetarian and nonvegetarian elderly women," *International Journal of Sports Medicine* 10(4) (1989): 243–251.

NIH Consenses Conference. "Triglyceride, High-Density Lipoprotein, and Coronary Heart Disease," *Journal of the American Medical Association* 269(4) (1993): 505–510.

"Nonpharmacological approaches to the control of high blood pressure. Final report of the subcommittee on nonpharmacological therapy of the 1984 Joint National Committee on Detection, Education, and Treatment of high blood pressure," *Hypertension* 8(5) (1986): 444–467.

Noren, K. "Levels of organochlorine contaminants in human milk in relation to the dietary habits of the mothers," *Acta Paediatrica Scandinavica* 72(6) (1983): 811–816.

Null, Gary. *The New Vegetarian.* New York, NY: Morrow, 1978.

Nutrition During Pregnancy. Washington D.C.: National Academy Press, 1990.

"Nutrition recommendations and principles for people with diabetes mellitus," *Journal of the American Dietetic Association* 94 (1994): 504–506.

Oberleas, D, and BF Harland. "Phytate content of food: effect on dietary zinc bioavailability," *Journal of the American Dietetic Association* 79(4) (1981): 433–436.

O'Connor, A. "Are Beef By-Products Risky?", *Vegetarian Times* 227 (1996): 16.

O'Connor, A. "Is BSE Just a British Problem?", *Vegetarian Times* 226 (1996): 16–17.

Ophir, O, et al. "Low blood pressure in vegetarians: The possible role of potassium," *American Journal of Clinical Nutrition* 37(5) (1983): 755–762.

Orlov, SN, et al. "Univalent cation fluxes in human erythrocytes from individuals with low or normal sodium intake," *Journal of Cardiovascular Risk* 1(3) (1994): 249–254.

Ornish, D, et al. "Can lifestyle changes reverse coronary heart disease?" *Lancet* 336 (1990): 129–133.

Packard, PT, and RP Heaney. "Medical nutrition therapy for patients with osteoporosis," *Journal of the American Dietetic Association* 97(4) (1997): 414–417.

Parachin, Victor. *365 Good Reasons to Be a Vegetarian: A Book of Thoughts, Facts, Humor, Science, and Surprises.* Garden City Park, NY: Avery Publishing Group, 1998.

Patterson, AG. "Now that soy protein has respect, how do you eat more?", *Soy Connection* 4(1) (1996): 2.

Patterson, AG. "Soy protein—additional defense against heart disease," *Soy Connection* 4(1) (1996): 2.

Peavey, BS, GF Lawlis, and A Goven. "Biofeedback-assisted relaxation: effects of phagocytic capacity," *Biofeedback & Self Regulation* 10(1) (1985): 33–47.

Pederson, AB, et al. "Menstrual differences due to vegetarian and nonvegetarian diets," *American Journal of Clinical Nutrition* 53(4) (1991): 879–885.

Peltonen R, et al. "Faecal microbial flora and disease activity in rheumatoid arthritis during a vegan diet," *British Journal of Rheumatology* 36(1) (1997): 64–68.

Pennington, J. *Bowes and Church's Food Values of Portions Commonly Used* (16th ed). Philadelphia, PA: JB Lippincott Company, 1994.

Persky, VW, et al. "Hormone levels in vegetarian and non-vegetarian teenage girls: potential implications for breast cancer tisk," *Cancer Research* 52(3) (1992): 578–583.

Peterson, C, et al. "Diet and Health Recommendations for Cancer Prevention," *American Institute for Cancer Research Newsletter* 58 (1998): 1, 3, 6–7.

Peterson, C, et al. "Where's the Meat? Some New Soy Options May Be Worth A Try," *American Institute for Cancer Research Newsletter on Diet, Nutrition and Cancer* 57 (1997): 6–7.

Phillips, RL, and DA Snowdon. "Dietary relationships with fatal colorectal cancer among Seventh Day Adventists," *Journal of the National Cancer Institute* 74(2): 307–317.

Pick, ME, et al. "Oat bran concentrate bread products improve long-term control of diabetes: A pilot study," *Journal of the American Dietetic Association* 96(12) (1996): 1254–1261.

Pixley, F, et al. "Effect of vegetarianism on development of gall stones in women," *British Medical Journal Clinical Research* 291(6487) (1985): 11–12.

Potter, JD. "Vegetables, Fruit, and Phytochemicals," *Soy Connection* 4(2) (1996): 1.

Potter, Norman. *Food Science.* New York, NY: Avi Books, Van Nostranol Reinhold, 1986.

Prineas, RJ, et al. "Walnuts and serum lipids," *New England Journal of Medicine* 329 (1993): 359.

Pringle, Lawrence. *Our Hungry Earth: The World Food Crisis.* New York, NY: Macmillan Co., 1976.

Pronczuk, A, Y Kipervarg, and KC Hayes. "Vegetarians have higher plasma alphatocopheral relative to cholesterol than do nonvegetarians," *Journal of the American College of Nutrition* 11(1) (1992): 50–55.

Proulx, WR, and CM Weaver. "Calcium absorption from plants," *Soy Connection* 2(2) (1997): 1, 4.

Raicht, RF, et al. "Protective effect of plant sterols against chemically induced colon tumors in rats," *Cancer Research* 40(2) (1980): 402–405.

Rauma, AL, et al. "Vitamin B_{12} status of long-term adherents of a strict uncooked vegan diet ('living food diet') is compromised," *Journal of Nutrition* 125(10) (1995): 2511–2515.

Reddy, S, TA Sanders, and O Obeid. "The influence of maternal vegetarian diet on essential fatty acid status of the newborn," *European Journal of Clinical Nutrition* 48(5) (1994): 358–368.

Reed, JA, et al. "Comparative changes in radical bone density of elderly female lacto-ovovegetarians and omnivores," *American Journal of Clinical Nutrition* 59(suppl) (1992): 1197s–1202s.

"Relationship between the calcium-to-protein ratio in milk and the urinary calcium excretion in healthy adults: A controlled crossover study," *American Journal of Clinical Nutrition* 52(1) (1990): 142–146.

Repetto, R. "Renewable Resources and Population Growth," *Population and Environment* 10(4) (Summer, 1989): 228–229, cited in Rifkin's *Beyond Beef* (New York: Dutton Press, 1992).

Resnicow, K, et al. "Diet and serum lipids in vegan vegetarians: A model for risk reduction," *Journal of the American Dietetic Association* 91 (1991): 447–453.

Retta, TM, GM Afre, and OS Randall. "Dietary management of blood pressure," *Journal of the Association for Academic Minority Physicians* 5(4) (1994): 147–151.

Reuters. *Year After Gene Controversy—US Milk Consumption Up* (Jan 31, 1995).

Richter, A, et al. "Morphological and morphometric measurements in colorectal mucosa of subjects at increased risk for colonic neoplasia," *Cancer Letters* 74(1–2) (1993): 65–68.

Rifkin, J. *Beyond Beef: The Rise and Fall of the Cattle Culture*. New York, NY: Plume, 1993.

Ritter, MM, and WO Richter. "Effects of a vegetarian life style on health," *Fortschr Der Medicine* 113(16) (1995): 239–242.

Robbins, J. *Diet for a New America*. Walpole, NH: Stillpoint Publishing, 1987.

Robbins, J. *May All Be Fed: Diet for a New World*. New York, NY: William Morrow & Company, Inc., 1992.

Robertson, L, C Flinders, and B Ruppenthal. *The New Laurel's Kitchen: A Handbook for Vegetarian Cookery and Nutrition*. Berkeley, CA: Ten Speed Press, 1986.

Rolfes, SR, and LK DeBruyne. *Life Span Nutrition: Conception Through Life*. St. Paul, MN: West Publishing Company, 1990.

Rosellini, L. "How far should you go to stay fit? The battle between tough and tame," *U.S. News & World Report* 123(18) (1997): 95–96.

Rouse, IL, et al. "Blood-pressure-lowering effect of a vegetarian diet: Controlled trial in normtensive subjects," *Lancet* 1(8314-5) (1983): 5–10.

Rouse, IL, et al. "Vegetarian diet, lifestyle, and blood pressure in two religious populations," *Clinical and Experimental Pharmacology and Physiology* 9 (1982): 327–330.

Rouse, IL, BK Armstrong, and LJ Beilin. "The relationship of blood pressure to diet and lifestyle in two religious populations," *Journal of Hypertension* 1(1) (1983): 65–71.

Rouse, IL, and LJ Beilin. "Vegetarian diet and blood pressure," *Journal of Hypertension* 2(3) (1984): 231–240.

Row, DA. "History of Promotion of Vegetable Cereal Diets," *Journal of Nutrition* 116 (1986): 1355–1363.

Runners World (June, 1992): 66.

Sabate, J, et al. "Does nut consumption protect against ischemic heart disease?", *European Journal of Clinical Nutrition* 47(suppl 1) (1993): 571–545.

Sabate, J, et al. "Attained height of lacto-ovo vegetarian children and adolescents," *European Journal of Clinical Nutrition* 45(1) (1991): 51–58.

Sabate, J, et al. "Effects of walnuts on s-lipid levels and blood pressure in normal men," *New England Journal of Medicine* 328(9) (1993): 603–607.

Sabate, J, MC Llorca, and A Sanchez. "Lower height of lacto-ovovegetarian girls at preadolescence: an indicator of physical maturation delay?", *Journal of the American Dietetic Association* 92(10) (1992): 1263–1265.

Safina, C. "The World's Imperiled Fish," *Scientific American* (Nov, 1995).

Sanchez, A, et al. "Changes in levels of cholesterol associated with plasma amino acids in humans fed plant proteins," *Nutrition Reports International* 32 (1985): 1047–1056.

Sanders, TA. "Good nutrition for the vegetarian mother," *Modern Midwife* 4(4) (1994): 230–236.

Sanders, TA, et al. "Studies of Vegans: The fatty acid composition of plasma choline phosphoglycerides, erythrocytes, adipose tissue, and breast milk and some indicators of susceptibility to ischemic heart disease in vegans and omnivore controls," *American Journal of Clinical Nutrition* 31(5) (1978): 805–813.

Sanders, TA, FR Ellis, and JW Dickerson. "Haematological studies on vegans," *British Journal of Nutrition* 40(1) (1978): 9–15.

Sanders, TA, S Reddy. "The influence of a vegetarian diet on the fatty acid composition of human milk and the essential fatty acid status of the infant," *Journal of Pediatrics* 120 (1992): s71–74.

Sanders, TA, S Reddy. "Vegetarian diets and children," *American Journal of Clinical Nutrition* 59(suppl) (1994): 1176s–1181s.

Sanders, TA, and F Roshanai. "Platelet phospholipid fatty acid composition and function in vegans compared with age- and sex-matched omnivore controls," *European Journal of Clinical Nutrition* 46(11) (1992): 823–831.

Santos, ML, and DA Booth. "Influences on meat avoidance among British students," *Appetite* 27(3) (1996): 197–205.

Schuler, G, et al. "Regular physical exercise and low-fat diet. Effects on progression of coronary artery disease," *Circulation* 86(1) (1992): 1–11.

Schneider, W, and E Menden. "The effect of long-term increased protein administration on mineral metabolism and kidney function in the rat. II. Kidney function and bone mineralization," *Zeitschrift fur Ernahrungswissenschaft* 27(3) (1988): 186–200.

Sciarrone, SE, et al. "Ambulatory blood pressure and heart rate responses to vegetarian meals," *Journal of Hypertension* 11(3) (1993): 277–285.

Sciarrone, SE, et al. "Biochemical and neurohormonal responses to the introduction of a lacto-ovovegetarian diet," *Journal of Hypertension* 11(8) (1993): 849–860.

Science News 150 (Sept 14, 1996): 173.

Scrimshaw, NS, CE Taylor, and JE Gorden. "Interactions of nutrition and infection," *Nutrition* 4 (1988): 13–50.

Seiler, D, et al. "Effects of long-distance running on iron metabolism and hematological parameters," *International Journal of Sports Medicine* 10(5) (1989): 357–362.

Sharma, DC, and R Mathur. "Correction of anemia and iron deficiency in vegetarians by administration of ascorbic acid," *Indian Journal of Physiology & Pharmacology* 39(4) (1995): 403–406.

Sharma, V, and Sharma A. "Serum cholesterol levels in carcinoma breast," *Indian Journal of Medical Research* 94 (1991): 193–196.

Shaw, NS, CJ Chin, and WH Pan. "A vegetarian diet rich in soybean products compromises iron status in young students," *Journal of Nutrition* 125(2) (1995): 212–219.

Shibatta, A, et al. "Intake of vegetables, fruits, beta-carotene, vitamin C and vitamin supplements and cancer incidence among the elderly: A prospective study," *British Journal of Cancer* 66(4) (Oct, 1992): 673–679

Shils, Maurice E., ed. *Modern Nutrition in Health and Disease* (8th ed). Lea & Febiger, 1994.

Shrapnel, WS, et al. "Diet and coronary heart disease: The National Heart Foundation of Australia," *Medical Journal of Australia* 1156 (suppl) (1992): 59–61.

Shultz, TD, and JE Leklem. "Vitamin B_6 status and bioavailability in vegetarian women," *American Journal of Clinical Nutrition* 46(4) (1987): 647–651.

Siddiqui, MK, et al. "Chlorinated hydrocarbon pesticides in blood of newborn babies in India," *Pesticides Monitoring Journal* 15(2) (1981): 77–79.

Siguel, EN. "Cancerostatic effect of vegetarian diets," *Nutrition and Cancer* 4(4) (1983): 285–291.

Simon, JA. "Ascorbic acid and cholesterol gallstones," *Med-Hypotheses* 40(2) (1993): 81–84.

Sirtori, CR. "Soy protein and cholesterol reduction: From infancy to old age," *Soy Connection* 4(2) (1996): 2.

Sizer, Frances, and Eleanor Whitney. *Nutrition: Concepts and Controversies.* Belmont, CA: Wadsworth Publishing Company, 1997.

Slavin, JL. "Health benefits of soy fiber," *Soy Connection* 3(2) (1995): 1.

Slavin, J, J Lutter, and S Cushman. "Amenorrhoea in vegetarian athletes," *Lancet* 1(8392) (1984): 1474–1475.

Snow, P, and K O'Dea. "Factors affecting the rate of hydrolysis of starch in food," *American Journal of Clinical Nutrition* 34 (1981): 2721–2727.

Snowdon, DA, and RL Phillips. "Does a vegetarian diet reduce the occurrence of diabetes?", *American Journal of Public Health* 75(5) (1985): 507–512.

Snowdon, DA, RL Phillips, and GE Fraser. "Meat consumption and fatal ischemic heart diseases," *Preventative Medicine* 13(5) (1984): 490–500.

Snowdon, DA, and P Roland. "Does a vegetarian diet reduce the occurrence of diabetes?", *American Journal of Public Health* 75(5) (1984): 507–512.

Snyder, AC, LL Dvorak, and JB Roepke. "Influence of dietary iron source on measures of iron status among female runners," *Medicine & Science in Sports & Exercise* 21(1) (1989): 7–10.

So, F, et al. "Inhibition of human breast cancer cell proliferation and delay of mammary tumorigenesis by flavonoids and citrus juices," *Nutrition and Cancer* 26(2) (1996): 167–181.

Sobel, BS. "Cut the fat, cut the risk: A low-fat diet can reduce your risk of breast cancer," *Total Health* (1994): 12.

Soy Connection 5(1) (1997): 3.

Spake, Amorda. "O is for Outbreak," *U.S. News & World Report* 123(20) (1997): 70–84.

Specker, BL. "Nutritional concerns of lactating women consuming vegetarian diets," *American Journal of Clinical Nutrition* 59 (suppl) (1994): 1182s–1186s.

Specker, BL, et al. "Effect of vegetarian diet on serum 1,25-dihyfroxyvitamin D concentrations during lactation," *Obstetrics & Gynecology* 70(6) (1987): 870–874.

Spencer, H, L Kramer, and D Osis. "Factors contributing to calcium loss in the aging," *American Journal of Clinical Nutrition* 36 (Oct, 1982): 776–787.

Spiller, GA, DJA Jenkins, et al. "Effects of a diet high in monounsaturated fat from almonds on plasma cholesterol and lipoproteins," *Journal of American College of Nutrition* 11 (1992): 126–130.

Sri-Kantha, S, and JW Erdman Jr. "Legume carotenoids," *Critical Review of Food Science Nutrition* 126(2) (1987): 137–155.

St. Jeor, ST, et al. *(1995) Nut Consumption and Its Correlates in the RENO Diet Heart Study.* San Fransisco, CA: USDA-ARS Western Human Nutrition Center, Presidio of San Francisco, September, 1995.

Stahelin, HB, et al. "Beta-carotene and cancer prevention: The Basel Study," *American Journal of Clinical Nutrition* 53 (1991): 2655s–2659s.

Stammers, JP, et al. "High arachidonic acid levels in the cord blood of infants of mothers on vegetarian diets," *British Journal of Nutrition* 61 (1989): 89–97.

Stampfer, NJ, et al. "A prospective study of plasma homocysteine and risk of myocardial infarction," *Journal of the American Medical Association* 268 (1992): 877–881.

Stauber, John. "Apocalypse Cow," *PR Watch,* First Quarter 3(1) (1996).

Steinberg, D, and workshop participants. "Antiosicants in the prevention of human atherosclerosis," *Circulation* 85(6) (1992): 2338.

Stollholf, K, and FJ Schulte. "Vitamin B_{12} and brain development," *European Journal of Pediatrics* 146(2) (1987): 201–205.

Stone, Sally, and Martin Stone. *The Instant Bean.* New York, NY: Bantam Books, 1996.

Stoy, DB, et al. "Cholesterol-lowering effects of ready-to-eat cereal containing psyllium," *Journal of the American Dietetic Association* 93(8) (1993): 910–912.

Sugano, M, et al. "Cholesterol-lowering activity of various undigested fractions of soy bean protein in rats," *Journal of Nutrition* 120 (1990): 977–985.

Sullivan, KH. "The Iron File," *Vegetarian Times* 227 (1996): 58–65.

Suzuki, H. "Serum vitamin B_{12} levels in young vegans who eat brown rice," *Journal of Nutritional Science & Vitaminology* 41(6) (1995): 587–594.

Szabo, L. "The health risks of new-wave vegetarianism," *Canadian Medical Association Journal* 156(10) (1997): 1454–1455.

Tanaka, T, et al. "Chemoprevention of organs carcinogenesis by natural product protocatechuic acid," *Cancer* 75(suppl 6) (1995): 1433–1439.

Tayler, M, and KL Stanek. "Anthropometric and dietary assessment of omnivore and lacto-ovovegetarian children," *Journal of the American Dietetic Association* 89(11): 1661–1663.

Taylor, CB, et al. "Serum cholesterol levels of Seventh Day Adventists," *Paroi Arterielle* 3(4) (1976): 175–179.

Tesar, R, et al. "Axial and peripheral bone density and nutrient intakes of postmenopausal vegetarian and omnivorous women," *American Journal of Clinical Nutrition* 54(4) (1992): 699–704.

Thomas, J, and FR Ellis. "The health of vegans during pregnancy," *Proceedings of the Nutrition Society* 36(1) (1977): 46A.

Thorogood, et al. "Risk of death from cancer and ischaemic heart diseases in meat and non-meat eaters," *British Medical Journal* 308(6945) (1994): 1667–1670.

Toniolo, P, et al. "Consumption of meat, animal products, protein, and fat and risk of breast cancer: a prospective cohort study in New York," *Epidemiology* 5(4) (Jul, 1994): 391–397.

Toohey, ML, et al. "Cardiovascular disease risk factors are lower in Afro-American vegans compared to lacto-ovo vegetarians," *Journal of the American College of Nutrition* 17(5) (1998): 425–434.

"Trans-Fatty Acids and Serum Cholesterol Levels," *Nutrition Reviews* 49(2) (1991): 57–60.

Treuherz, J. "Zinc and dietary fiber: observations on a group of vegetarian adolescents," *Proceedings of the Nutrition Society* 39(1) (1980): 10A.

Trichopoulou, Antonia, et al. "Consumption of olive oil and specific food groups in relation to breast cancer risk in Greece," *Journal of the National Cancer Institute* 87(2) (1995): 110–116.

Trichopoulou, D, et al. "Diet and cancer of the stomach: A case-control study in Greece," *International Journal of Cancer* 36 (1985): 290–297.

Trinchieri, A, et al. "The influence of diet on urinary risk factors for stones in healthy subjects and idiopathic renal calcium stone formers," *British Journal of Urology* 67(3) (1991): 230–236.

Tufts University Health & Nutrition Letter 16(8) (Oct, 1998): 1.

Tylavsky, FA, and JB Anderson. "Dietary factors in bone health of elderly lactoovovegetarian and omnivorous women," *American Journal of Clinical Nutrition* 48 (1988): 842–849.

United States General Accounting Office. *Rangeland management: Comparison of rangeland condition reports.* Report to the Chairman, Subcommittee on National Parks and Public Lands, Committee on Interior and Insular Affairs, House of Representatives. Washington, DC: US GAO, 1991. (GAO/RCED–91–191).

United States General Accounting Office. *Rangeland management: Forest Service not performing needed monitoring of grazing allotments.* Report to the Chairman, Subcommittee on National Parks and Public Lands, Committee on Interior and Insular Affairs, House of Representatives. Washington, DC: US GAO, 1991. (GAO/RCED–91–148).

Urivetzky, M, et al. "Dietary protein levels affect the excretion of oxalate and calcium in patients with absorptive hypercalciuria type II," *Journal of Urology* 137(4) (1987): 690–692.

Urjman, N, et al. "Diet, nutrition intake, and metabolism in populations at high and low risk for colon cancer. Metabolism of bile acids," *American Journal of Clinical Nutrition* 40 (suppl 4) (1984): 937–941.

US Department of Agriculture. "Crops: Area, Yield, Production, and Value, United States, 1986–1999," *Agricultural Statistics 1989* (table 554, pg. 390). U.S. Department of Agriculture. Washington, DC: GPO, 1989.

US Department of Health and Human Services. *Diet, Nutrition, & Cancer Prevention: A Guide to Food Choices.* Washington, DC: U.S. Department of Health and Human Services, Public Health Service, National Institutes of Health (NIH Publication No. 87-2878), revised May 1987.

US Department of Health and Human Services. *Healthy People 2000: National Health Promotion and Disease Prevention Objectives.* Washington, DC: US Department of Health and Human Services, Public Health Service, 1991 (DHHS publication PHS 91-50212).

US Department of Health, Education, and Welfare. *Healthy People: The Surgeon General's Report on Health Promotion and Disease Prevention.* Washington, DC: US Department of Health, Education, and Welfare, 1979.

US Dietary Guideline Committee, US Department of Agriculture, and US Department of Health and Human Services. "Nutrition and Your Health: Dietary Guidelines for Americans (4th ed)," *Home & Garden Bulletin* 232 (1995).

USDA Report. "BSE Rendering Policy" (1991), in John Stauber's *Apocalypse Cow, PR Watch*, First Quarter 3(1) (1996).

Van de Weerdt, DH. "Contamination of production animals with environmental pollutants and public health risk (abstract)," *Tijdschrift voor Diergeneeskunde* 117(19) (1992): 554–558.

Van-Faassen, A, et al. "Bile acids and pH values in total feces and in fecal water from habitually omnivorous and vegetarians subjects," *American Journal of Clinical Nutrition* 58(6) (1993): 917–922.

Vegetarian Resource Group. Survey in *Vegetarian Journal* (July/Aug, 1994).

Wachman, A, and DS Bernstein. "Diet and osteoporosis," *Lancet* 1 (1968): 958–959.

Walter, P. "Effects of vegetarian diets on aging and longevity," *Nutrition Reviews* 55(1, pt 2) (1997): s61–65.

Wasserman, Debra, and Reed Mangels. *Simply Vegan: Quick Vegetarian Meals.* Vegetarian Resource Group, 1999.

Watson, RR. "Immunological enhancement by fat-soluble vitamins, minerals, and trace metals: A factor in cancer prevention," *Cancer Detection and Prevention* 9(1–2) (1986): 67–77.

Weaver, CM, and KL Plawecki. "Dietary calcium: adequacy of a vegetarian diet," *American Journal of Clinical Nutrition* 59(suppl 5) (1994): 1238s–1241s.

Wedling, T. "Diners have no way to know if restaurant food is safe to eat," *Plain Dealer* (Nov 9, 1997): 1–A, 14–A.

Weekly, SJ. "Diets and eating disorders: Implications for the breastfeeding mother," *NAACOGL Clinical Issues in Perinatal & Women's Health Nursing* 3(4) (1992): 695–700.

Weisburger, JH. "Dietary fat and risk of chronic diseases: mechanistic insights from experimental studies," *Journal of the American Medical Association* 97(suppl) (1997): S16–S23.

Weisburger, JH. "Mechanism of action of diet as a carcinogen," *Cancer* 43(suppl 5) (1979): 1987–1995.

Welch, RM, and JW Findlay. "Excretion of drugs in human breast milk," *Drug Metabolism Reviews* 12(2) (1981): 261–277.

Wenger, NK, L Speroff, and B Packard. "Cardiovascular health and diseases in women," *New England Journal of Medicine* 329(4) (1993): 247.

West, BB, and L Wood. *Foodservice in Institutions* (6th ed). New York, NY: Macmillan Publishing Company, 1988.

West, KM, and JM Kalbfleisch. "Influence of nutritional factors on prevelance of diabetes," *Diabetes* 120 (1971): 99–108.

West, RO, and OB Hayes. "Diet and Serum Cholesterol Levels: A Comparison Between Vegetarians and Nonvegetarians in a Seventh-day Adventist Group," *American Journal of Clinical Nutrition* 21(8) (1968): 853–862.

Westrich, BJ. "Effect of physical activity on skeletal integrity and its implications for calcium requirement studies," *Nutrition and Health* 5(1–1) (1987): 53–60.

White, Ellen G. *Counsels for the Church.* Boise, ID: Pacific Press Publishing Association, 1991.

White, Ellen G. *Ministry of Healing.* Boise, ID: Pacific Press Publishing Association, 1905.

Whitney, EN, CB Cataldo, and SR Rolfes. *Understanding Normal Clinical Nutrition* (3rd ed). St. Paul, MN: West Publishing Company, 1991.

Whorton, JC. "Historical Development of Vegetarianism," *American Journal of Clinical Nutrition* 59(suppl 5) (1994): 1103s–1109s.

Willett, WC, et al. "Mediterranean diet pyramid: A cultural model for healthy eating," *American Journal of Clinical Nutrition* 61 (suppl 6) (1995): 1402s–1406s.

Willett, WC, et al. "Micronutrients and cancer risk," *American Journal of Clinical Nutrition* 59(suppl) (1994): 1162s–1165s.

Willett, WC, et al. "Relation of meat, fat, and fiber intake to the risk of colon cancer in a prospective study among women," *New England Journal of Medicine* 323 (1990): 1664–1672.

Willett, WC, et al. "Weight, weight change and coronary heart diseases in women—risk within the normal weight range," *Journal of the American Medical Association* 273(6) (1995): 461–463.

Williams, C. "Healthy eating: clarifying advice about fruit and vegetables," *British Journal of Nutrition* 310 (1995): 1453–1455.

Williams III, G. "What's wrong with fish?", *Vegetarian Times* 216 (1995): 54–59.

Winter, R. *Poisons in Your Plate.* New York, NY: Crown Publishers, Inc., 1969.

Wolman, PG. "Management of patients using unproven regimens for arthritis," *Journal of the American Dietetic Association* 87(9) (1987): 1211–1214.

Woodruff, Sandra. *Secrets of Cooking for Long Life.* Garden City Park, NY: Avery Publishing Group, 1999.

Wootan, M, and B Liebman. "The Great Trans Wreck," *Nutrition Action Healthletter* (1993): 10–12.

"World Health Organization-sponsored workshop on Lactose Malabsorption (Moscow, June 10–11, 1985)," in "National Dairy Council, Nutritional implications of lactose and lactase activity," *Dairy Council Digest* 56 (1985): 25–30.

Wright. "The Fifth Report of the Joint National Committee on Detection, Evaluation, and Treatment of High Blood Pressure (JNC V)," *Archives of Internal Medicine* 153 (1993): 154–162.

Wright. "National High Blood Pressure Education Program Working Group Report on Primary Prevention of Hypertension," *Archives of Internal Medicine* 153 (1993): 186–208.

Young, VR, and PL Pellett. "Plant proteins in relation to human protein and amino acid nutrition," *American Journal of Clinical Nutrition* 59(suppl) 1994: 1203s–1212s.

Index